Physiotherapy in Rheumatology

SYLVIA A. HYDE

MCSP

Superintendent Physiotherapist
Hammersmith Hospital, and
Royal Postgraduate Medical School, London

With contributions by

O.M. SCOTT MCSP
R.E. JARVIS MCSP
R.A. HARRISON MCSP

BLACKWELL SCIENTIFIC PUBLICATIONS

OXFORD LONDON EDINBURGH
BOSTON MELBOURNE

LONDJ(NN) GLG

© 1980 by
Blackwell Scientific Publications
Editorial offices:
Osney Mead, Oxford, OX2 0EL
8 John Street, London, WC1N 2ES
9 Forrest Road, Edinburgh, EH1 2QH
52 Beacon Street, Boston, Massachusetts 02108,
    USA
214 Berkeley Street, Carlton
    Victoria 3053, Australia

First published 1980

DISTRIBUTORS

USA
    Blackwell Mosby Book Distributors
    11830 Westline Industrial Drive
    St. Louis, Missouri 63141
Canada
    Blackwell Mosby Book Distributors
    120 Melford Drive, Scarborough
    Ontario, M1B 2X4
Australia
    Blackwell Scientific Book Distributors
    214 Berkeley Street, Carlton
    Victoria 3053

British Library
Cataloguing in Publication Data
Hyde, Sylvia A
    Physiotherapy in rheumatology.
    1. Arthritis   2. Rheumatism
    3. Physical therapy
    I. Title
    616.7′2   RC933
    ISBN 0-632-00373-1

Set by Typesetting Services Ltd., Glasgow
printed in Great Britain by Morrison & Gibb Ltd.

Physiotherapy in Rheumatology

Contents

Contributors

Mrs O. M. Scott MCSP
Research Physiotherapist
Physiotherapy Department
Hammersmith Hospital
London

Mrs R. E. Jarvis MCSP
Superintendent Physiotherapist
Canadian Red Cross Memorial Hospital
Taplow

R. A. Harrison MCSP
Superintendent Physiotherapist
Royal National Hospital for Rheumatic Diseases
Bath

Foreword

Despite the exacting professional training in physiotherapy, the subject, like a number of medical specialities, has often been criticised for its traditionalism and lack of scientific enquiry. Many of the time-hallowed forms of therapy—some would say the majority—have not been put under the controlled scrutiny expected of medical or surgical procedures.

Happily this situation is changing quickly, and many units, notably that at the Hammersmith, under the leadership of Sylvia Hyde, are actively combining therapy and research. Throughout this book, the thoughtful and modern approach taken by Mrs Hyde and her team shows through. Reading the proofs of this volume has been a pleasure. The book gives a clear and up-to-date description of the major rheumatic diseases and the present role of the physiotherapist in treatment. It also indicates, in no uncertain way, that physiotherapy is a science.

G. R. V. Hughes, MD, FRCP
Head of Rheumatology Unit,
Royal Postgraduate Medical School

Preface

This book helps student physiotherapists to understand the principles of treatment of those diseases broadly encompassed by the term rheumatology. The inclusion of some references and quantitative methods of measuring muscle output both stimulates and assists the qualified physiotherapist to look afresh at the physical management of this group of patients. The increasing knowledge of the role of immunological processes in this complex group of diseases is rapidly modifying both classification of disease entities and their management. The physiotherapist must, therefore, consult modern texts for current developments that may have implications for physiotherapy.

Inevitably an author writes within the framework of experience, and it is accepted that the detailed physiotherapy is greatly influenced by the referring rheumatologist and, therefore, only the principles and rationale of treatment are explored. Emphasis is placed on assessment and serial measurement because in these diseases, characterised by an erratic and unpredictable course, each patient must be treated as an individual. The long term, and often chronic, nature of the disease has such far reaching effects on the patient's physical well-being and social fabric that a team approach to management is essential.

In the preparation of this book I have been greatly assisted by many people. Mr D. Simmonds and Mr D. Hawtin contributed the excellent clinical illustrations. Dr G. R. V. Hughes and his colleagues have given invaluable support and his personal enthusiasm has been an inspiration. Mrs O. Scott's contribution has been inestimable both as clinician and researcher. My sincere thanks go to all of them.

I would also like to thank all the physiotherapy staff at Hammersmith, in particular Miss J. Brown, for their constructive criticism of the manuscript and their support during its preparation, without which it would not have been completed.

To Miss J. L. Morris, my predecessor and constant mentor, my gratitude.

S.A.H.
JULY 1979

1 Introduction and Classification

Rheumatoid arthritis is but one of a large group of diseases in which polyarthritis or arthralgia, inflammatory changes and pain are the predominant features. The end effect of these changes on patient mobility and dexterity are often so profound that they cause significant alterations in the patient's social, economic and occupational status. It is estimated that at least one person in twenty is affected by the disease during his life and the literature abounds with demographic studies illustrating the effect of this disease on industry and the national economy. The practice of rheumatology is not concerned only with rheumatoid arthritis but with a complex group of diseases that in addition to affecting the musculoskeletal system manifest multisystem symptoms. Improved laboratory techniques and an increased understanding of immunology and the immune complex system have vastly increased the potential for differential diagnosis within the group, so that separate disease entities continue to emerge.

Classification of the many separate diseases, embraced by the term rheumatological, has proven difficult, as indeed has the nomenclature. The classification below has wide acceptance and is used for clarity.

Nomenclature and classification of the rheumatic diseases

1. Polyarthritis of unknown aetiology:
   Rheumatoid arthritis
   Still's disease
   Ankylosing spondylitis
   Psoriatic arthropathy

2. Connective tissue disorders:
   Systemic lupus erythematosus
   Polyarteritis nodosa
   Progressive systemic sclerosis
   Polymyositis
   Dermatomyositis
3. Rheumatic fever
4. Degenerative joint disease:
   Primary
   Secondary
5. Non-articular rheumatism
6. Diseases with which arthritis is frequently associated
7. Associated with known infectious agents
8. Traumatic and/or neurogenic disorders:
   Syringomyelia
   Shoulder hand syndrome
9. Associated with known biochemical or endocrine abnormalities:
   Haemophilia
   Gout
10. Tumour and tumour-like conditions of joints
11. Allergy and drug reactions
12. Inherited and congenital disorders
13. Miscellaneous disorders:
   Osteochondritis desicans
   Tietze's disease

The group of diseases broadly embraced by the term polyarthritis of unknown aetiology may be further subdivided on the basis of response to serological testing for rheumatoid factor.

The importance of definitive diagnosis in a group of diseases where, for the most part, the aetiology and pathogenesis remain unknown may at first sight seem of more academic interest than clinical significance but it is of importance both in determining therapy and in attempting prognosis.

Traditionally, patients with rheumatological disorders have been referred for rehabilitation and predominantly physiotherapy. Unfortunately, in the past, all too frequently, the therapeutic objective has simply been palliation of pain and provision of aids to mobility, the presence of active joint disease and pain appearing to contraindicate active physical measures. Both physiotherapist and patients had, therefore, to accept the chronic state and what seemed to be the inevitable decline. Physiotherapy cannot cure the arthritis but physical measures can prevent or retard deterioration in the musculoskeletal system and preserve or enhance the patient's locomotor ability and independence. Skilful and thoughtful application of physiotherapy techniques demands an accurate, quantitative and complete assessment of the patient's locomotor system.

The physiotherapist can only determine the best physical treatment programme if she has an understanding of the disease process and relates physiotherapeutic measures to this. In the chapters that follow an attempt has been made to relate the physiotherapy aims and objectives to the pathology. Hence, the account of the pathological changes and clinical features has been scantily attacked except where it is of significance to the physiotherapist.

Haematology, serology and muscle enzyme studies are similarly only referred to as they affect the prescription of physiotherapy and a résumé of these tests is given in Appendix A. The importance of the development of immunology and the relevance of this to understanding the connective tissue diseases have already been alluded to but any attempt at discussion of the immune system would be inappropriate. The reader is, therefore, referred to Hughes, G. R. V. (1977) *Connective Tissue Diseases*, Ch. 14. Blackwell Scientific Publications, Oxford.

2 Muscle and Exercise

The physiotherapist in clinical practice spends much of her time working with patients who have disorders of muscle; this dysfunction may be the result of primary involvement of muscle tissue, or secondary to involvement of other systems. The acceptance of the concept that exercise can change and improve muscle function is central to treatment by physical means.

It is, therefore, pertinent that the physiotherapist has an understanding of the effect of exercise on muscle and indeed on the other systems of the body. The development of an effective and appropriate exercise programme for any given patient will be dependent on the physiotherapist's ability to integrate her knowledge of the physiology of muscle and exercise with functional anatomy within the framework of the underlying pathology.

The detailed architecture and microstructure of muscle is found in the available texts, so that here it is only necessary to review the basic components.

Sarcolemma. This is the surface membrane of the muscle fibre.

Muscle fibres. These are composed of myofibrils each consisting of the protein myofilaments – actin and myosin.

There are two main types of muscle fibre (Fig. 2.1a, b):

Type I (*red*). These are rich in the mitochondrial oxidative enzymes used in carbohydrate metabolism and fatty acid oxidation. They have a higher concentration of mitochondria and myogloblin which serves as an oxygen store. Type I fibres rely upon aerobic metabolism within

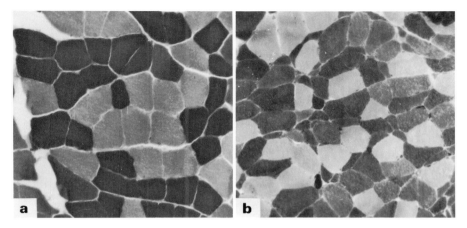

Fig. 2.1. Cross section of (a) normal skeletal muscle showing Type I (light fibre) and Type II fibres; and (b) Skeletal muscle showing atrophy of Type I fibres from disuse. ATPase 9.4 × 250 (courtesy of C. Maunder and Dr A. Young).

the mitochondria for energy source. Type I fibres have a slower contraction time and are therefore more suited to sustained work.

Type II (*white*). These fibres are larger than Type I fibres, have high concentrations of glycogen and phosphorylase and rely upon anaerobic glycolysis within the sarcoplasm for energy source. They are more suited to quick activity. Type II fibres are further sub-divided into three groups on the basis of histochemical staining but so far the functional importance of these subgroups has not been demonstrated.

Excitation–contraction coupling

Muscular contraction occurs as a result of a series of events involving interaction of electrophysiological, biochemical and mechanical forces.

Failure at any stage in the complicated chemical system, or defect in the structure of the muscle, will result in ineffectual contraction or changed indices of contraction, for example, speed of contraction or relaxation.

MUSCLE FUNCTION

The normal function of a muscle is to produce tension which is appropriate to the demand. Strength is synonymous with tension, and is normally recorded as the maximum tension that can be produced by voluntary effort. It is necessary to look at the relationship between maximum tension and varying length of the muscle (Fig. 2.2). In static contraction, that is where there is no movement of the joint over which the muscle works but there is some muscle shortening to take up slack, maximum tension has been shown to develop at a length about 10% greater than the resting length. The maximum contractile tension reaches its lowest at full length and full shortening [1].

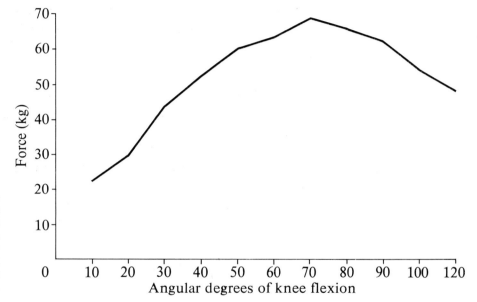

Fig. 2.2. The relationship between the angle of the knee joint measured from full extension and the maximum voluntary force output of the right quadriceps femoris muscle.

In contractions where joint motion occurs with lengthening or shortening of the muscle (isotonic, concentric–eccentric) the maximum point of tension occurs at a length near the resting length.

Other factors that mediate the tension that a muscle can develop are:

1. Motivation and voluntary effort
2. The integrity of the central nervous system
3. The degree of synaptic inhibition

Methods of testing muscle function

Until recently methods of testing muscle function were concerned only with measuring the force output of muscle contracting at the subject's volition, or with measuring the muscle's ability to sustain a contraction for a given time [2]. In practice it is usually torque that is measured. This is the rotation produced around a joint, which depends on the angle of pull of the muscle and the length of lever; in this case the distance between the attachment of the muscle and the axis of movement of the joint (Fig. 2.3). All these methods are dependent on, or influenced by, other factors, for example, motivation and muscle mass. Muscle bulk has been measured and taken as an index of muscle strength for centuries but it is really an index of potential strength.

Methods developed more recently [3] have made it possible to supplement the more traditional methods of testing muscle. Using electrical stimulation, so by-passing volitional control, it is now possible to describe muscle function in terms of:

1. Force/frequency curve: the relative forces produced by different frequencies of stimulation.
2. Speed of relaxation.
3. The ability to sustain tension during prolonged stimulation.

Normal values for these indices have been established.

These methods of measuring muscle function are, as yet, not widely

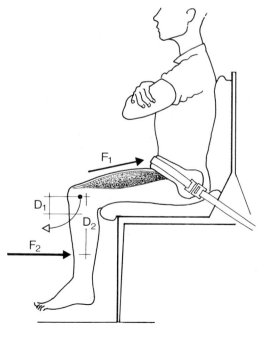

Fig. 2.3. Chair used for measuring muscle output. Torque $= F_1 \times D_1 = F_2 \times D_2$. F_1. Force output of quadriceps femoris muscle. D_1. Distance from axis of knee joint to attachment of quadriceps femoris. F_2. Force exerted against measuring bar. D_2. Distance from axis of knee joint to bar.

used but are invaluable in identifying specific abnormalities in muscle contractility and have been used in our department as a method of looking at the effect of exercise [4].

Exercise

Exercise can be defined as purposeful motion. Many systems of the body are involved in exercise and the ability to perform efficiently depends not only on the integrity of each system but also on their successful integration and ability to work together. Throughout any activity the various body systems are required to adapt to changing needs. There is a vast internal control system which co-ordinates the response to the increased demands, regulating the output of the circulatory and respiratory systems, balancing temperature regulation, in addition to the specific response of the neuromuscular system.

In the musculoskeletal system the adaptation may be more permanent. Different types of exercise with regard to load, frequency, intensity and co-ordination will produce different changes in the muscle, and it is essential in planning physical treatment to identify what changes or adaptations are desired. Training is a method of systematic increased exercise demand by loading and is performed to raise the level of overall fitness/function of the individual. It is the concept of the body's ability to adapt and in particular the ability of muscle to adapt, that is the basis of therapeutic exercise.

The aim of training is to reduce the overall energy cost, to balance the metabolic capacity and to increase mechanical efficiency. A further discussion of the factors affecting metabolic capacity, bloodflow, oxygen uptake, and cardiac output would not be appropriate here, but the interested reader can turn to the standard texts on the subject.

It is however important to note that an exercise programme designed to improve overall muscle power and physical fitness must:

1. Be of sufficient intensity and duration to raise cardiac output to near maximum;
2. Be of sufficient intensity to utilise anaerobic mechanisms;
3. Tax local and general circulation by using large muscle groups.

Power

This implies the performance of work in a definite period of time.

$$\text{Muscle power} = \frac{\text{Work}}{\text{Time}}$$

In exercise, work is done by shortening muscle and energy is required for the sliding of the actin filaments between the myosin and the formation of cross bridges.

Nearly all chemical processes are exogenic and resting muscle releases energy as heat to the environment. During isometric contraction, more heat is liberated than at rest. It has been shown [5] that when muscle contracts isotonically it does Work,

$$\text{Work} = \text{Force} \times \text{Distance}$$

where the Force is the load supported by the contracting muscle and Distance is the distance through which it is moved.

Fatigue

This brief résumé of muscle structure, its response to different demands and the specific adaptations that different forms of exercise demand, would not be complete without mention of fatigue, particularly since it is so often of concern in the management of rheumatological disorders.

Fatigue may be general, general physical or local muscular in origin. In general fatigue, psychological factors such as lack of motivation and interest play a part as well as the body's physiological response. General physical fatigue is thought to be a state of disturbed homeostasis [6]; however, relatively little is known about the mechanism by which this occurs.

Local muscular fatigue occurs as a result of the muscle's depletion of energy stores, the factors influencing this being blood flow and type of muscle contraction. The necessary energy for short bursts of isometric exercise can be obtained from adrenotriphosphate and phosphocreatine and if the workload is less than 15% of maximum, the blood supply of oxygen is sufficient for the muscle to work aerobically for long periods. If the contraction is maximal, fatigue will occur rapidly because the blood supply is markedly reduced and hence the oxygen supply, and the muscle is then dependent upon anaerobic processes for the release of energy (Fig. 2.4).

The controversy about the role of the central nervous system, and in particular the synapses in fatigue has continued over many years. It is now generally accepted that fatigue of muscle results from energy depletion rather than synaptic blocking [7].

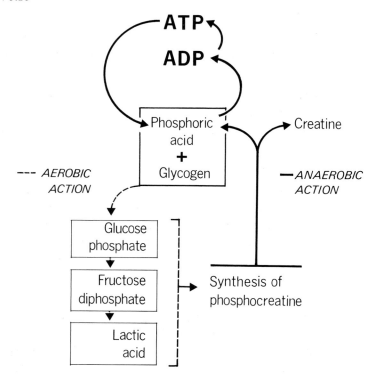

Fig. 2.4. Schematic representation of energy source for muscle contraction.

EXERCISE PROGRAMMES

The design of an appropriate exercise programme for a rheumatological patient will, therefore, take into consideration the following:

1. The change or adaptation required in the muscles:
    a. Improved strength/force output
    b. Ability to sustain force output – reduction of fatigue at local level
2. The disease entity and its manifestations:
    a. Muscle involvement: Type I or Type II muscle fibre
    b. Joint involvement: the effect of movement on joints with regard to irritability, pain, effusion
    c. Soft tissue involvement: the effect of tension, stretching on ligaments, capsules and tendons
    d. Other systems: cardiac, respiratory, metabolic
3. Overall level of fitness

4. Functional level: the need for improvement in activities of daily living

5. The need for improvement of joint range of motion.

Physiotherapists commonly describe exercise in terms of the type of movement evoked, namely assisted, free and resisted. The method of applying the resistance varies and may be manual or by the use of apparatus such as weights, springs or torque devices.

Free exercise

In this form of exercise a series of movements are performed without assistance or resistance being introduced. The exercise may be performed simply to maintain the range of motion of a particular joint or may be done as part of a fitness training programme, in which case the parameters of time and frequency are introduced.

Resisted exercise

The core of physiotherapy and in particular the restoration of muscle strength depends upon the understanding of the mechanics of muscle contraction outlined in this chapter. The number of fibres in a given muscle does not vary much from one individual to another, and it would appear that the restoration of muscle function depends on adequate loading of the muscle so that it contracts with maximum or near maximum force.

It is our experience that in the clinical situation in the management of the rheumatological diseases, where pain, contractures and positioning are significant factors, the use of manual resistance is the method of choice in the application of resistance or load to the muscle. Techniques of proprioceptive neuromuscular facilitation [8] afford the opportunity to load the muscle maximally throughout range without placing stress on the joints (Fig. 2.5). Pain and fatigue are also kept to a minimum when these techniques are skilfully applied.

Skill or control exercises

Motor learning is repetitive, amply demonstrated by the normal maturation of locomotor activity. The newborn infant moves in response to a series of stimuli and only later, as development proceeds, are the mass reflex motor responses sublimated and segmented so that

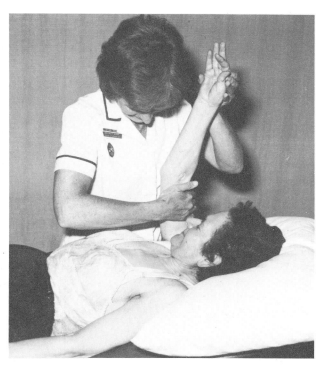

Fig. 2.5. Manual resistance exercise using flexion abduction external rotation with repeated contractions for shoulder abductors.

volitional, purposeful movements are achieved. Purposeful movement, e.g. turning, standing, walking, is only attained after each component of the movement has been repeated many times.

That further training of skilled movement is possible in the fully developed normal adult is demonstrated by the skills acquired in occupation and sport. It has been shown that it is possible to train subjects to fire single motor units [9]. The further development or acquisition of control (co-ordination, smoothness of response) is obviously not concerned with muscle alone but with the training or enhancement of the central nervous system as well.

Exercise as a means of improving range of movement

Physiotherapists frequently use exercise as a method of restoring or improving range of motion of a joint or joints. Although the adaptation or response sought here is not primarily one of muscle but of local connective tissue and ligamentous structures it is appropriate to discuss these methods.

Smooth range of motion requires that the agonist has sufficient strength to move the lever arm, that the antagonist relaxes and the fulcrum of movement (i.e. the joint) is not constrained by limiting factors such as adhesions or ineffectual joint lubrication. The properties of the synovial fluid, the response of the molecular structure of this under stress and the effect of movement on the nutrition of cartilage are well documented.

In the rheumatological disorders a significant factor in restricting range of motion is pain-induced muscle spasm. Only in the later stages of the disease are ligamentous and capsular contractures the major feature. Hold-relax and contract-relax techniques [8] are most beneficial in restoring range of motion.

In summary the contractile properties of muscle have been reviewed, the types of exercise in relation to work performed discussed and an attempt made to correlate these with the prescription and definition of therapeutic exercise programmes. In the rheumatological disorders where loss of muscle power is frequently observed, together with muscle wasting and poor physical fitness, it is important for the physiotherapist to clearly define the objectives of an exercise programme in relation to these deficiencies.

REFERENCES

[1] ASMUSSEN E. (1962) Muscular performance. In *Muscle as a Tissue*, ed. by Rodahl K. and Horvath S. M. McGraw-Hill, New York.
[2] FESSEL W. J., TAYLOR J. A. & JOHNSON E. S. (1970) In *Muscle Diseases*, p. 544, ed. by Walton J. L., Canal L. and Scarlato G. Amsterdam.
[3] EDWARDS R. H. T., YOUNG A., HOSKING G. P. & JONES D. A. (1977) Human skeletal muscle function: description of tests and normal values. *Clinical Science and Molecular Medicine*, **52**, 283–290.
[4] GRAHAM O. & HYDE S. A. (1978) Clinical application of quantitative muscle testing. *8th International Congress, World Confederation for Physical Therapy*.
[5] FENN W. O. & MARCH B. S. (1935) Muscle force at different speeds of shortening. *Journal of Physiology*, **85**, 277–297.
[6] CHRISTENSEN E. H. (1962) Muscular work and fatigue. In *Muscle as a Tissue*, ed. by Rodahl K. and Horvath S. M. McGraw-Hill, New York.
[7] MERTON P. A. (1954) Voluntary strength and fatigue. *Journal of Physiology*, **123**, 553–564.
[8] KNOTT M. & VOSS D. E. (1968) *Proprioceptive Neuromuscular Facilitation Techniques*. Harper and Row, London.
[9] BASMAJIAN J. V. (1963) Control and training of individual motor units. *Science*, **141**, 440–441.

FURTHER READING

ASTRAND P.-O. & RODAHL K. (1977) *Textbook of Work Physiology*. McGraw-Hill, New York.
CARLSÖÖ S. (1972) *How Man Moves*. Heinemann, London.
RODAHL K. & HORVATH S. M. (1962) *Muscle as a Tissue*. McGraw-Hill, New York.

3 Examination and Assessment

The patient who presents in the physiotherapy department with a diagnosis of one of the rheumatological disorders has already had a thorough examination by the doctor. The examination will have included the following basic components:

1. History of complaint
2. Physical examination
3. Laboratory tests
4. Radiological examination

The purpose of the examination is to establish a diagnosis based on the findings and to determine a therapeutic programme.

The physiotherapist's examination of the patient, which must be equally thorough, is to provide:

1. Information to determine the best method of physical treatment
2. Baseline data to monitor subsequent therapy, e.g. physical, drug therapy
3. Information that will be helpful to other members of the team caring for the patient

The examination includes objective and subjective tests and some which are a mixture of both.

The rheumatological disorders affect many tissues and joints so it is necessary to examine the whole patient, although only one joint may manifest overt signs of the disease.

It is essential to consider the physical and social changes in the whole person both in evaluation of the problem and in subsequent treatment planning.

It is not always necessary to undertake the whole assessment at follow-up visits but simply to select one or two parameters.

It is most helpful to adopt a systematic method of examination, as this will decrease the chance of overlooking important points. However, some flexibility is needed, as there are those patients who, presenting with single joint involvement, will be upset that primary attention is not given to that joint. It is also important to explain carefully to the patient the reason for the examination and method. The depth and framework in which the explanation is given depends upon the patient's understanding of the disease. It is important that good dialogue exists between members of the team and that the rheumatologists' attitudes to patient education are known.

The physiotherapist examines the patient making observations of the following:

1. General:
    a. Gait analysis
    b. Skin changes
    c. Temperature
2. Pain
3. Swelling
4. Muscle power
5. Joint range
6. Deformity
7. Respiratory function
8. Functional capacity
9. Functional assessment – activities of daily living.

The methods used to examine and measure the above are numerous, and the method finally adopted in any unit may depend on the availability of equipment, manpower resources, philosophy of management and previous experience. It is certain that, unlike the measurement of lung function, for example, there is not one 'right' way and indeed in many areas of the examination there is not one internationally accepted unit of measurement. In the following paragraphs methods of examination and assessment are described which the author has found useful, but for the benefit of the reader examples of other methods are given and where appropriate the merits of each discussed.

RECORDING

It is essential that the findings of the examination are recorded clearly and concisely and are easily retrievable. The record should be intelligible to other members of the team of experts caring for the patient. The following should be noted:

Rheumatoid disease has a natural history which often spans several decades, with periods of exacerbation and remission. It is therefore essential that serial measurements are made.

1. Unit of measurement
2. Starting position
3. Time of day
4. Day of week
5. Factors influencing measurements obtained:
   a. Change in drug therapy
   b. Period of exercise
   c. Concurrent illness

GENERAL OBSERVATIONS

Gait analysis

Ideally the physiotherapist should be able to observe the patient walking without him being aware of it; skilful observations made at this time will act as cues during the more formal examination. It also provides an opportunity to observe the natural walking pattern.

1. Aids if used
2. Trendelenburg's sign (positive or negative)
3. Lateral shift of trunk
4. Weight acceptance
5. Push off
6. Swing through
7. Cadence
8. Width of base
9. Rhythm
10. Symmetry

It is helpful to observe these features in the same order each time.

Skin changes

Is the skin thin and transparent?
  Are there skin lesions present?

1. Psoriatic
2. Disproportionate subcutaneous haemorrhages (Fig. 3.1)
3. Nail bed lesions, denoting arteritis (Fig. 3.2)
4. Skin changes typical of a neurological involvement
5. Changes in skin elasticity

Temperature

Skin temperature and any excess sweating of the hands should be assessed.

Differences in temperature over joints are noted by placing the dorsal aspect of the examining hand alternately over the joint being tested and over the same joint on the opposite limb. Care of course is taken to ensure that the subtle difference perceived is not the result of a bandage that has just been removed.

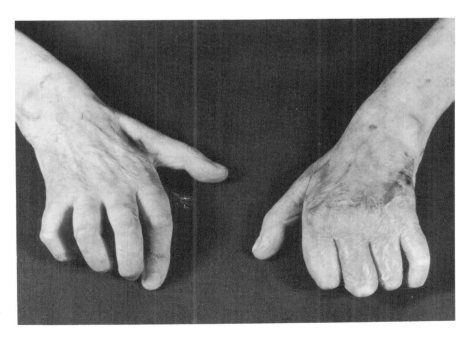

Fig. 3.1. Shows subcutaneous haematomas on dorsum of left hand and typical skin changes in a patient with sero positive rheumatoid arthritis. Atrophy of the interossei is evident.

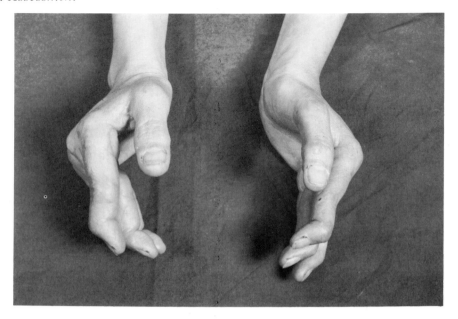

Fig. 3.2. Nail bed lesions in patient with arteritis.

PAIN

The perception of pain and the physical and emotional response to pain are unique to each individual. If a patient declares that he has pain, he has, regardless of whether the examiner can find an attributable physical cause.

The objective measurement of pain and the understanding of the pain mechanism has puzzled clinicians and research workers for many decades. The hypothesis of the gate mechanism [1] has extended our knowledge of pain production and pain perception considerably, but as yet there is no entirely objective method of quantitating pain. Rather we rely upon subjective methods.

Two methods are described which have been found useful clinically.

Method I

The patient is given a sheet of paper on which there is drawn a six inch line, with only the ends of the line labelled, at one end no pain and at the other extreme pain. The patient is then asked to draw a parallel line, stopping where he perceives his pain to be in relation to the two extremes.

No pain ————————————————— Extreme pain

The examiner is able to plot a graph from information so gained.

Method II

The patient is asked to grade his pain.
Grade I   – no pain
    II – some pain
    III – moderate pain
    IV – severe pain

The exploration of pain has so far been entirely the patient's account, i.e. subjective; now the examiner attempts gently to elicit pain.

Is there (a) pain on pressure?
      (b) pain on passive movement?
      (c) pain on active movement?

If so, (a) where is the site of the pain?
      (b) when does the pain occur, i.e. at what part of the range of movement?

The examiner uses a knowledge of anatomy to interpret the findings and localise the structure causing pain.

Pain on pressure

This is tested by applying direct pressure with the pulps of the fingers and gradually increasing the pressure. In this way the structure causing the pain may be accurately localised.

Pain on passive movement

The joint to be examined is carefully put through full passive range of all its physiological movements. Compression of the joint at the same time will give added information and help to differentiate between those problems arising from intra-articular disease and extra-articular problems. In the acute rheumatoid joint there will be pain throughout the range.

Pain on active movement

This may be from involvement of tendons or muscles, or the effect of increasing the pressure in an already distended joint. The point at which pain is felt will be helpful in differentiation.

SWELLING

Swelling around a joint is indicative of tissue reaction to disease process but a knowledge of the exact nature of the swelling and the structures involved is important to the physiotherapist. The swelling may be either soft tissue swelling or fluid. Careful reflection on the anatomical arrangement of the joint being examined, together with palpation, can differentiate between intra-articular and extra-articular swelling and determine the nature of that swelling. The synovium of the rheumatoid joint produces a swelling that has a characteristically 'boggy' feel and in advanced disease the synovium may feel thickened (Fig. 3.3). Where there is fluid within a joint, it may be fluctuated across the joint by the examiner's hands. Calcinosis or new bone formation has a characteristic hard feel.

It is helpful, although not entirely reliable, to compare the joint

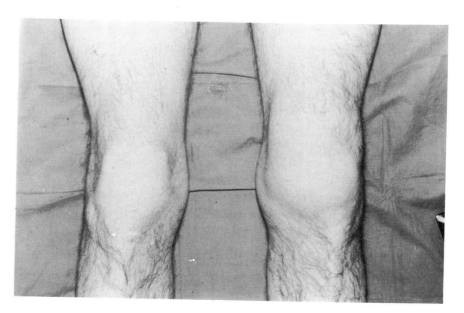

Fig. 3.3. Synovial effusion of left knee in patient with rheumatoid arthritis.

being examined with the one on the opposite side. To measure swelling of the finger joints a jeweller's ring size is used, whilst for larger peripheral joints a tape measure suffices, but in either case bony landmarks must be located.

Where more than one joint in a limb is involved or where there is gross swelling, volume displacement methods may be used. In routine clinical practice the latter method is rarely necessary, except perhaps with hands.

MUSCLE POWER

Measurement of muscle power is universally done using the MRC scale. This scale, as every physiotherapist knows, grades the power of individual muscles from 0–5 using standardised positions. There are, nevertheless, problems with this method of assessment, namely that the severely involved patient, or one in an acute phase of the disease, is often unable to achieve the standard position for the test. Secondly the method of grading is partially subjective, so that one frequently finds inter-observer differences to the extent that plus or minus signs are used, e.g. 3+ may be recorded as 3 by another observer. It must also be remembered that, in normal function, muscles do not work individually but in groups. The scale is only able to reflect gross changes in muscle power.

The degree of accuracy that is required will be determined by the patient's pathology. For example in the patient with rheumatoid arthritis it is often sufficient to use the MRC scale for muscle groups but in patients with polymyositis it may well be necessary to measure more accurately.

It is worthy of comment that as early as 1916 attempts were made to introduce objective methods of muscle testing and since then there have been many endeavours to bring into clinical usage numerous devices to measure and record muscle power. Unfortunately, those most closely involved with rehabilitation have been reluctant to adopt objective methods of quantitation, and such devices have been reserved for research projects and trials. An excellent review of methods of quantitation is to be found in communications from the Testing and Observation Institute, Denmark [2].

Perhaps one reason why dynamometers (sometimes called myometers when specifically designed to measure muscle) have not found favour with clinicians is that many of them are bulky pieces of apparatus, requiring a source of power to operate, and are expensive.

However, for some patients, we prefer to supplement the MRC scale with measurements of muscle force using a dynamometer. There are many such devices available commercially, each with their own merit. Here only the Hammersmith dynamometer [3] will be described in detail (Fig. 3.4a, b).

It is a small hand-held device that is small enough to fit conveniently in the pocket when not in use. The dynamometer comprises an oil filled bellows and a pressure gauge. The force exerted is directly proportional to the pressure, since the cross section of the bellows remains constant. The force exerted is recorded in newtons.

Standardised positions are used both for the starting position of the muscle group to be tested and for placement of the dynamometer. Bony points are used for siting the dynamometer. The force recorded is that which the examiner needs to exert to overcome the patient's maximum contraction. It is usual to take the best of three readings.

Muscle wasting

Loss of muscle bulk is only an indication of muscle attrition and is not a good or reliable index of the muscle's ability to generate force. This was demonstrated by a trial undertaken at Hammersmith Hospital in 1957 [4]. A tape measure is used and circumferential measurements are made from bony landmarks and compared with the opposite limb.

JOINT RANGE

It is necessary to measure active and passive movement and note any difference between the two ranges.

Joint range of motion is measured and recorded according to the method described by the American Academy of Orthopaedic Surgeons in 1965 [5].

A simple goniometer is used but the importance of accurate localisation of fixed bony landmarks and the use of a suitable size of goniometer cannot be overstressed. For large joints such as the hip, knee and elbow, in an average adult, a goniometer with 12 inch arms is recommended whilst for smaller joints such as the finger a $1\frac{1}{2}$ inch goniometer arm is needed.

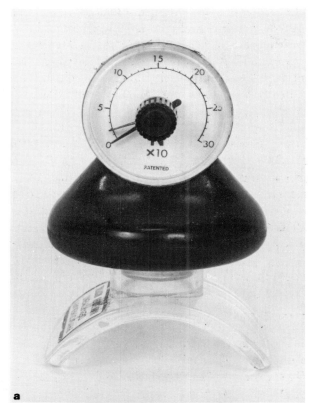

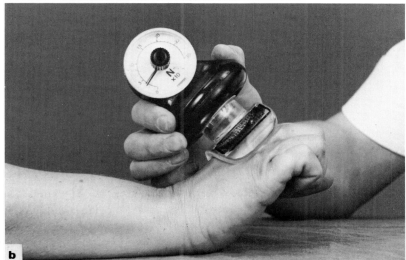

Fig. 3.4. (a)
Hammersmith
myometer; (b) Testing
wrist extensors using
myometer.

The metacarpophalangeal and interphalangeal joints may also be measured using thin lead strips. These strips are very malleable and are placed over the joint and bent to fit the contour of the joint. The bent lead strip is then placed on paper and a line drawn parallel to the edge, the angle being measured using a protractor, or the angle is drawn on graph paper. This method is particularly helpful where serial measurements are made and provides a graphic illustration of the finger.

Spinal movement

It is rarely necessary to measure spinal movement in the rheumatological disorders, the exception being ankylosing spondylitis; details of spinal measurement techniques are therefore found in Chapter 9.

The hand

This requires special mention, because its function is so complex, being dependent on the integrity of many small joints and the delicate, precise interaction of many muscles. The hand is integral to the patient's functional ability in activities of daily life and vital to quality of life. It is usual to assess the hand considering the four basic abilities, grip, power, pinch and apposition; particular care is essential in standardising positions (Fig. 3.5).

The following methods are used for hand assessment:

Dynamometers

These are usually devices using strain gauges and are often used to measure pinch grip, apposition and the force exerted by individual digits.

Grip strength (Fig. 3.6)

This is a semi-objective measurement of the power the hand exerts and is easily measured using a sphygmomanometer cuff that is folded and sewn to a suitable size and inflated to a pressure of 20 mmHg. The position for measurement is standardised; the patient sits with the elbow supported, the forearm in neutral with the elbow at 90° flexion. The patient then squeezes the cuff achieving a maximum grip. The best of three readings is used.

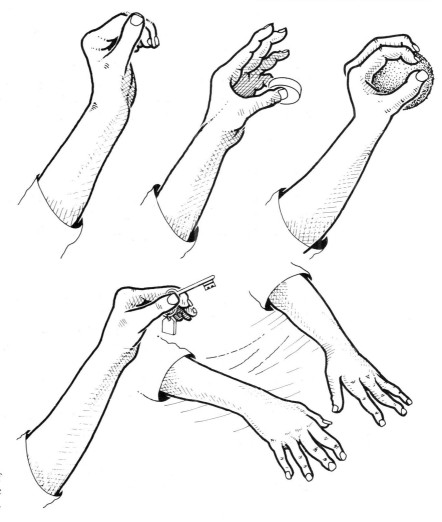

Fig. 3.5. Assessment of hand function – basic grips.

Wynthrop torquometer

It is possible to measure torque using this device but studies [6] have demonstrated good correlation between grip strength and torquometry, so that there is little advantage in measuring both.

Grip strength has also been shown to provide an index of pain and good correlation has been found [7] between the patient's subjective assessment of pain and grip strength.

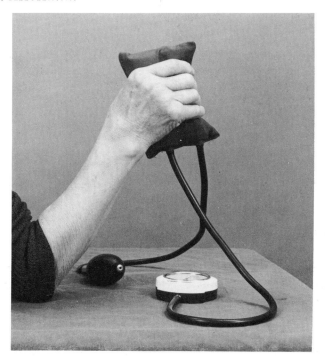

Fig. 3.6. Grip strength measurement, note the position of forearm in mid position pronation/supination, elbow supported at 90° flexion.

Volume displacement methods

This is useful where there is gross swelling.

Photography

This is done using standard positions. Where one is recording an active movement, rather than static position, a simple line drawing illustrating the movement attempted is included in the photograph.

Plaster casts

The primary disadvantage of this method is the space required to store the moulds.

DEFORMITY

The presence of deformity is noted and the deformity described and measured as in joint motion.

JOINT INSTABILITY

This is usually measured or estimated by the doctor or surgeon but it is necessary for the physiotherapist to note the presence of joint instability because this influences the rehabilitation programme (Fig. 3.7a, b).

RESPIRATORY FUNCTION

Vital capacity and forced expiratory volume (FEV_1) are measured.

FUNCTIONAL CAPACITY

This is a measurement of the patient's ability to perform physiological work (see p. 8). It reflects a combination of muscle power, metabolism, cardiovascular and respiratory function. The simplest index is walking time. This is the time, measured in seconds, taken to walk a fixed distance. Various other exercise tolerance tests using treadmills, measuring oxygen uptake etc. are described by physiologists but these are not used routinely in clinical work.

FUNCTIONAL ASSESSMENT

In this chapter, so far, only the clinical examination has been discussed. This will provide the physiotherapist with an indication of:

1. General disease activity
2. Local joint disease activity
3. Degree of deformity and consequent functional instability
4. Degree of involvement of extra-articular structures

However, if realistic and purposeful rehabilitation goals and treatment programmes are to be formulated it is essential that an index of the patient's functional level is made. Isolated measurements of muscle power and joint range are meaningful to neither the patient nor the therapist, and it is only when these are related to an activity of daily living that a total assessment of the patient can be said to have been made.

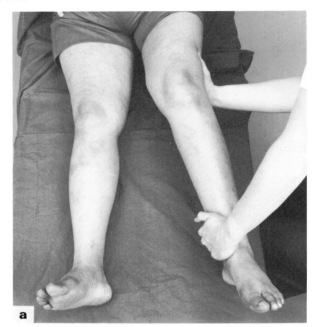

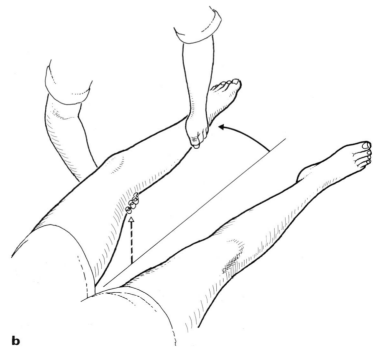

Fig. 3.7. (a) Examination for medial instability of the knee. (b) The knee is in slight flexion to relax the anterior cruciate ligament, the tibia is abducted on the femur.

Functional assessment will include aspects of:

1. Mobility
2. Dexterity
3. Personal care
*4. Home conditions
*5. Recreational activities
*6. Work

The use of scales of functional assessment is widespread and varies between the use of a four or five point scale applied to a limited number of activities, and a comprehensive scale embracing sixty or more activities of daily living. Both extremes present difficulties to the clinician, the former only registering gross changes and the latter being time consuming.

An example of the shorter scale is the ARA criteria of function in which patients are assessed on their ability to cope with everyday activities and assigned to one of four groups. The advantage of this method is that formal testing procedures, using equipment, are not necessary.

Functional classes – ARA [8]

I   Complete ability to perform all usual activities without handicap
II Normal activities adequate despite discomfort or limited motion of one or more joints
III Limited only to little or none of the duties of usual occupation or self care
IV Largely or wholly incapacitated. Bedridden or confined to wheelchair, little or no self care.

The above scale is not particularly helpful to the physiotherapist in defining the patient's exact functional deficit or assisting her to plan a treatment programme.

An index consisting of only seventeen questions that could be used by patient or clinician has been described [9]. The study demonstrated that the index had a high degree of inter- and intra-observer reproducibility. Other more detailed methods [10] of assessing functional level are used in some centres.

---

* Denotes those more commonly assessed by the occupational therapist, but in which the physiotherapist may contribute.

There are probably as many assessment charts in use as there are physiotherapy departments and this reflects the size of the problem. Some basic criteria for the design of assessment charts are:

1. Is the test reproducible?
2. Does it add to the information or simply duplicate?
3. Will it enhance treatment planning?
4. Is the method of scoring sufficiently sensitive?
5. Is the information easily retrievable?

REFERENCES

[1] MELZACK R. (1973) *The Puzzle of Pain*. Ch. 6, pp. 153–190. Penguin, Harmondsworth.
[2] ASMUSSEN E. (1959) Communications from the Testing and Observation Institute of the Danish National Association for Infantile Paralysis.
[3] EDWARDS R. H. T. & MCDONNELL M. (1974) Hand-held dynamometer for evaluating voluntary muscle function. *Lancet*, **ii**, 757–758.
[4] HAMILTON D. E., BYWATER E. G. L. & PLEASE N. W. (1959) A controlled trial of various forms of physiotherapy in arthritis. *British Medical Journal*, **i**, 542–544.
[5] AMERICAN ACADEMY OF ORTHOPAEDIC SURGEONS. (1965) *Joint Motion, Method of Measuring and Recording*.
[6] BREWER K., GUYALL A. R. & SCOTT J. T. (1975) Comparing grip strength. *Physiotherapy*, **61(4)**.
[7] INGPEN M. L. (1968) The quantitative measurement of joint changes in rheumatoid arthritis. *Annals of Physical Medicine*, **9**, 322–327.
[8] STEINBROCKER I., TRAEGER C. H. & BATTERMAN R. C. (1949) Therapeutic criteria in rheumatoid arthritis. *Journal of the American Medical Association*, **140**, 659–662.
[9] LEE P., JASANI M. K., DICK C. W. & BUCHANAN W. W. (1973) Evaluation of a function index in rheumatoid arthritis. *Scandinavian Journal of Rheumatology*, **2**, 71–77.
[10] LANSBURY J. (1968) Clinical appraisal of the activity index as a measure of rheumatoid activity. *Arthritis and Rheumatism*, **11**, 599–604.

4 Splinting and the Correction of Deformity

One of the most tragic and incapacitating manifestations of rheumatoid disease is the destruction of joints and tendons. The resultant loss of function is, together with pain, the commonest complaint of the patient presenting in the physiotherapy department. Adequate splintage and the use of orthoses and aids for ambulation can improve the patient's functional status.

Splints or orthoses are indicated for the following reasons:

1. Prevention of deformity
2. Correction of deformity
3. Prevention of trauma to an unstable joint
4. Improvement of function
5. Relief of pain

The physiotherapist usually makes those splints which are to be temporary, whilst the orthotist is responsible for permanent, formal orthoses. It is, nevertheless, essential that the physiotherapist is aware of the fundamentals of orthotics since in the care of the rheumatoid patient she will often be asked to advise on the type of appliance needed and will have to rehabilitate the patient using the appliance.

The materials commonly used by the physiotherapist are plaster of Paris, Prenyl, Plastazote, Orthoplast and Ortholast.

The choice of material is made after considering the physical properties of the material in relation to the forces, stresses and strains that it will be subjected to and the biomechanical function that the splint is to provide. Other factors are durability, ease of use and patient acceptance.

PREVENTION OF DEFORMITY

Rest splints

These splints are made, as the name suggests, to impose rest on the joint and are commonly worn at night. The joint is held in a neutral or optimum position and the splint should extend far enough on either side to stabilise it. If an over-corrected position is obtained the patient's acceptance of the splint is unlikely to be good because pain and spasm are evoked.

These splints are usually made of plaster of Paris and are carefully lined with lint.

The wrist and hand

Attention to the position of the carpometacarpal and metacarpo-phalangeal joints is essential, with the wrist in the optimum position in respect to radio-ulnar deviation, if the night splint is to be of benefit. The ideal position is one of function so that the wrist is held in approximately 25° extension, any ulnar deviation is corrected and the metacarpophalangeal joints are in minimal flexion. Care must be taken to ensure that the latter joints are not held in extension. If gross ulnar deviation of the fingers is present or if the patient is already showing signs of developing deformity, this is corrected by bridging the plaster to provide wedges; alternatively Plastazote spacers may be incorporated. Maintenance of the carpal arch is of vital importance.

If the thumb is included it is supported on the palmar aspect in slight extension and opposition.

The splint should extend from approximately three finger breadths below the ulnar head to the tips of the fingers (Fig 4.1a, b).

The knee

The most common deformity seen in rheumatoid disease is flexion contracture at the knee. A full length backslab of plaster of Paris is made and should extend from the level of the malleoli to the gluteal fold. When casting the knee it is helpful to have the patient in the prone position to obtain the maximum correction of the deformity. Care must be taken to ensure that the plaster extends sufficiently on

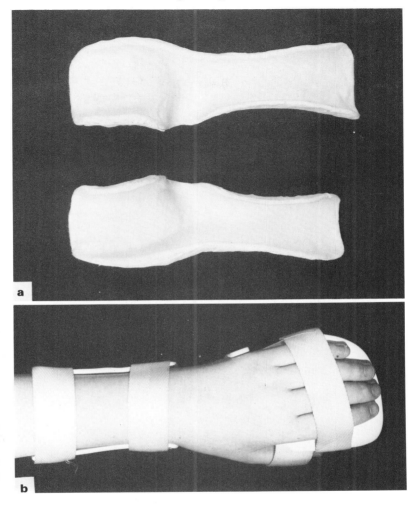

Fig. 4.1. (a) Rest splints for wrist (Hammersmith); (b) Paddle splints (courtesy of Canadian Red Cross Hospital).

the medial and lateral aspects to hold any valgus strain on the knee joint.

Plastazote is also used but is more likely to collapse and deform, so vitrathene reinforcement is incorporated, or a cylinder is made.

The foot and ankle

Where the ankle joint is also involved a foot piece is incorporated into the backslab to support the ankle in the plantagrade position and correct valgus or varus of the feet if present.

It must be remembered that the inclusion of the feet in the plaster is of great inconvenience to the adult who needs to visit the toilet at night, because it will necessitate removing the whole plaster.

CORRECTION OF DEFORMITY

Serial plasters

Serial plasters and stretch plasters are used to correct deformity. The integrity of the skin and circulation may be affected in rheumatoid arthritis and therefore caution and attention to pressure areas is of importance.

The knee

Serial plasters are made of plaster of Paris (Fig. 4.2a, b). A complete cylinder is made extending from malleoli to gluteal fold. To obtain maximum correction the patient should be treated immediately prior to the casting with ice packs and techniques of hold relax to the knee flexors and hip adductors. Traction is applied just above the malleoli and pressure exerted on the medial aspect of the knee joint to obtain maximum extension whilst the cast is made; it is inadvisable to exert direct pressure over the anterior aspect of the knee joint. Great care is taken in making the serial plaster to avoid pressure areas and it is helpful to place $\frac{1}{4}$ inch felt strips over the malleoli, knee joint and at the proximal end of the cast. (The patient should be carefully questioned to ensure that early signs of developing pressure areas are not overlooked and if in doubt the plaster is immediately removed.) The cast is then left for 48 hours before it is bivalved or split and hinged. The patient remains in the plaster, the cut edges having been tidied and smoothed, for several more days. The plaster is only removed for periods of intensive exercise to strengthen the quadriceps muscles. Once the patient can maintain the corrected position a new serial splint is made. The process is repeated until no further correction is obtained.

An alternative method of obtaining correction is by wedging the plaster. This is done by splitting the plaster horizontally over the posterior aspect of the knee joint, further extending the knee and then filling the gap with thin wedges of cork. These wedges are then held

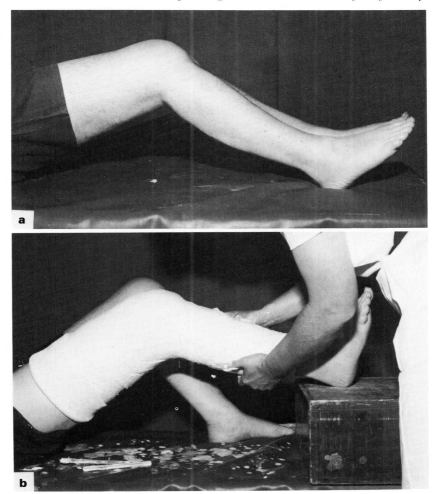

Fig. 4.2. (a) Knee flexion deformity in patient with rheumatoid arthritis; (b) Making serial plaster for the same patient.

in place with a few turns of plaster. If this method is used more padding should be placed over the anterior aspect of the knee when making the original cast.

The wrist

Serial splints are made for the wrist in the same manner as above. The plaster cylinder should not extend beyond the metacarpophalangeal joints, since it is unwise to attempt correction of more than one joint at a time.

Stretch plasters (Figs. 4.3, 4.4)

These are used primarily where there is tendon involvement and for small joints of the hand. Extreme stiffness of the interphalangeal and metacarpophalangeal joints is often found in scleroderma, systemic

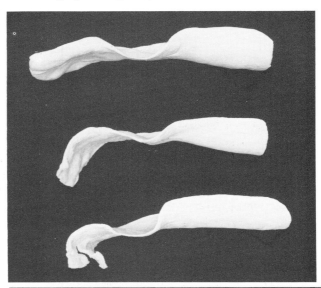

Fig. 4.3. Progression of stretch plasters.

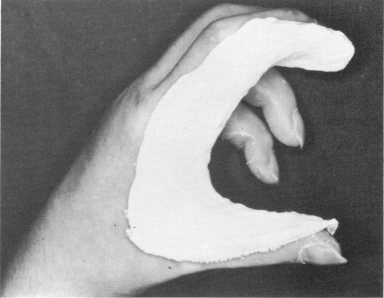

Fig. 4.4. Stretch plaster for web space in patient with scleroderma.

lupus erythematosus and in polyarteritis nodosa, due to flexor tendon tightness.

These plasters are used in rapid succession and detailed finishing is time-consuming and unnecessary.

PREVENTION OF TRAUMA TO AN UNSTABLE JOINT

There is considerable overlap between the use of splints to prevent trauma to an unstable joint and to improve function, the one often occurring as a consequence of the other. The biomechanical function that is required of the splint and the permanency of the device determines the type of splint and the material from which it is made (Fig. 4.5a, b). For example, in the lower extremity gross weakness of the quadriceps mechanism with some ligamentous laxity resulting in knee instability may necessitate temporary stabilising; an unstable wrist joint may require permanent splinting to improve hand function and relieve stress on the wrist joint.

The wrist

The *work splint* (Fig. 4.6) is provided to hold and protect the wrist joint in a functional position while allowing finger and thumb function. These splints are usually made of block leather or one of the plastic materials, the latter having the advantage of being washable. The wrist is held in 15°–25° extension but permits full movement at the metacarpophalangeal joints and first carpometacarpal joint. It is essential to check that pronation/supination in the splint does not cause pressure on the ulnar styloid. A further requirement of the work splint is that the patient is able to put the splint on without assistance. Velcro straps or closures are a considerable advantage.

Although there are many commercially available work splints these seldom provide the perfect fit that is necessary if adequate stabilisation is to be achieved and maximum enhancement of function obtained. It is apparent that without this patient acceptance is low.

The knee

In the case of the patient who has been non-ambulatory for some time and where the power of the quadriceps muscle is impaired, so that the

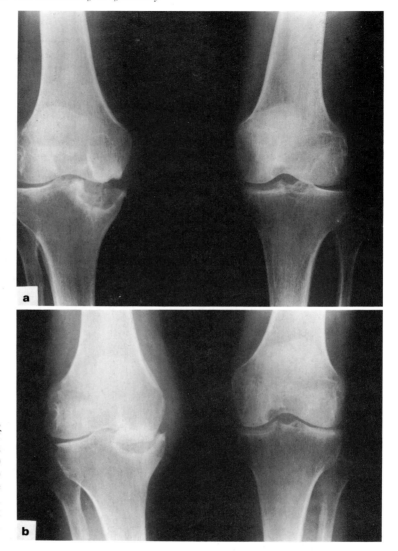

Fig. 4.5. Radiograph, anteroposterior view of knee in patient with rheumatoid arthritis. (a) Non weight bearing. (b) Weight bearing. Note the effect of compression on the joint space. A weight relieving caliper was used to improve function.

patient is unable to maintain the knees extended when walking, either a bivalved walking cylinder or a plaster backslab bandaged on is used to promote early ambulation.

Where the dual problem of residual knee flexion deformity or instability with quadriceps insufficiency is found, a walking cylinder is indicated. If the patient is in the early stages of rehabilitation and further correction of the knee with improved strength is sought, the

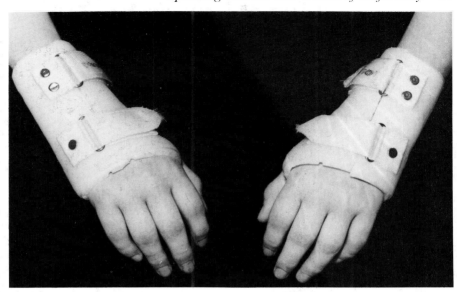

Fig. 4.6. Work splint for daytime use (courtesy of Canadian Red Cross Hospital, Taplow).

cylinder is made of plaster. However, where the knee remains unstable or where there is either flexion or valgus deformity in the presence of quadriceps weakness a more permanent cylinder is made of one of the hard plastic materials.

The spine

The cervical spine is frequently affected in rheumatoid disease and may present a life threatening situation if the odontoid process is eroded, causing pressure on the cord. In the more common manifestation of the disease the patient experiences all the signs and symptoms of cervical spondylosis with instability. The compression and wedging of vertebral bodies associated with prolonged high doses of corticosteroids is more commonly found in the thoracic and lumbar vertebrae and is seldom seen in the cervical spine.

Various types of collar are used and criteria for selection for an individual patient will depend on the degree of instability demonstrated.

1. Simple soft collar
2. Plastazote collar with front reinforcement of vitrathene to provide extension
3. Plastazote collar with jaw mould, anterior and posterior chest support (Fig. 4.7a, b). May also be made in polythene or Orthoplast.

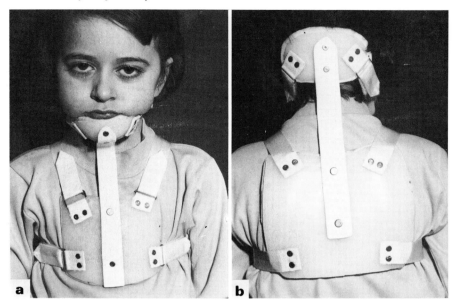

Fig. 4.7. Brace for control of neck and upper thoracic spine. (a) Front view. (b) Rear view. (Courtesy of Canadian Red Cross Hospital, Taplow.)

Lumbar and thoracic spine

Where there is collapse of vertebral bodies or pain from osteoporosis, early mobilisation is permitted by the use of temporary supports made from Plastazote. A spinal jacket is made with additional support being given by four 1 inch strips of vitrathene, two placed posteriorly just lateral to the spinal column and one in each mid-axillary line. By carefully moulding the Plastazote over the iliac crests the splint is prevented from riding up.

The foot and ankle

Splints for the foot and ankle are invaluable, often affording pain relief, improving mobility and preventing stress on the knee, hip and lumbar spine.

Plastazote shoes or boots are indicated as a temporary form of support for the acutely painful swollen foot. The painful heel syndrome, sometimes encountered in Reiter's disease or ankylosing spondylitis or in the presence of a calcaneal spur, is relieved by a doughnut-shaped rubber insert in the heel of the shoe. Plastazote insoles are also used as temporary arch supports or to relieve pressure on the metatarsal heads.

Cork is an excellent lightweight material for making temporary heel raises or heel and sole raises. The latter may be indicated where there is a leg length discrepancy resulting from contracture at the hip and knee; in these instances the cork raise can be serialised as the contracture decreases. Temporary cork raises may also be helpful in mobilising the restricted ankle joint.

Orthoses

The doctor prescribing an orthosis for his patient has identified the purpose of the orthosis and thus by implication has defined the biomechanical deficit demonstrated by the patient. The design and manufacture of the orthosis to fulfil that purpose and reduce the deficit is the task of the orthotist. The physiotherapist should be aware of the basic principles of orthotic prescription and of the various orthotic systems if she is to rehabilitate the patient successfully. She may also have a contribution to make in evaluating the orthosis during dynamic work.

Any orthosis should be re-evaluated at regular intervals to ensure that it continues to meet the patient's need and that it fits correctly.

The commonest orthoses used in the management of rheumatological disorders are the work splint, described on page 37, and orthoses to stabilise the knee and the ankle.

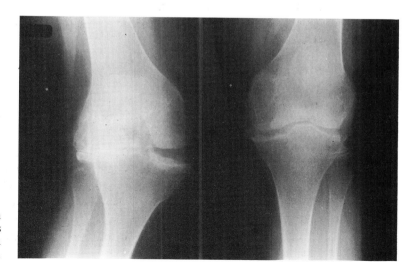

Fig. 4.8. Radiograph demonstrating valgus deformity in patient with rheumatoid arthritis.

In the unstable rheumatoid knee there are usually three components to be considered, flexion, valgus or varus and rotation (Fig. 4.8). In any brace there must be a three point contact to correct the deformity or control the forces tending to produce deformity. In the long leg standard caliper these points are the thigh band, the knee support and the shoe. In caliper construction the forces tending to produce valgus or varus are the most difficult to control and are most successfully controlled by the use of a pretibial shell (Fig. 4.9a, b). This effectively transmits the pressure over a much larger area and is therefore more comfortable than condylar pads.

The type of lock or hinge used at the knee joint is determined by the arc of movement which the patient is able to control voluntarily and the desired correction. Fixed knee flexion contracture is accommodated by offsetting the metal uprights distal to the knee joint. This may, however, produce a structural weakness in the brace.

Shoes

In the patient with painful and/or deformed feet the shoe becomes an important part of therapy and is prescribed with the same precision as drug therapy. The physiotherapist must become familiar with the various types of shoe and the modifications that can be made. In the re-education of gait and during subsequent re-assessments she must routinely check the patient's footwear. The shoe is prescribed either to achieve passive stabilisation and accommodate a severely deformed foot or to attempt active correction.

Moulded space shoes are an example of the former, with soft rubber soles and soft pliable leather uppers. These obviously have to be made from a cast of the patient's foot and are, like most custom-made appliances, expensive.

Good orthopaedic last shoes are adapted wherever possible, either externally or internally. Metatarsal pads, metatarsal bars, rockers, Thomas heels, etc, may be used. The range is extensive but each has a specific purpose (Fig. 4.10a, b).

In the discussion so far little emphasis has been placed on dynamic splinting, although it could be argued that some of the features in the long leg caliper just described are dynamic.

Dynamic splints are more frequently used for the hand and must be lightweight, easily adjustable and must enhance the patient's voluntary

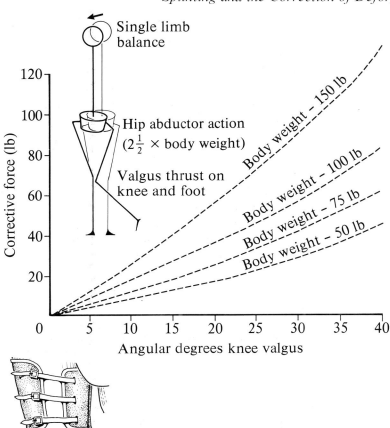

Single limb balance

Hip abductor action ($2\frac{1}{2}$ × body weight)

Valgus thrust on knee and foot

Body weight – 150 lb

Body weight – 100 lb

Body weight – 75 lb

Body weight – 50 lb

Corrective force (lb)

Angular degrees knee valgus

High medial flange to correct valgus deformity

Fig. 4.9. (a) Effect of weight as deforming force with progressive valgus deformity of the knee, and the force required for correction. (b) Pre-tibial shell. Arrow shows high medial flange to correct valgus deformity. Reprinted from *Principles of Lower Extremity Bracing* (1967) pp. 83 and 94, with the permission of the American Physical Therapy Association.

movement. They are used either to maintain constant stretch of soft tissue or to substitute for an action that the patient has lost. The provision of dynamic splints is often crucial to successful rehabilitation following hand surgery.

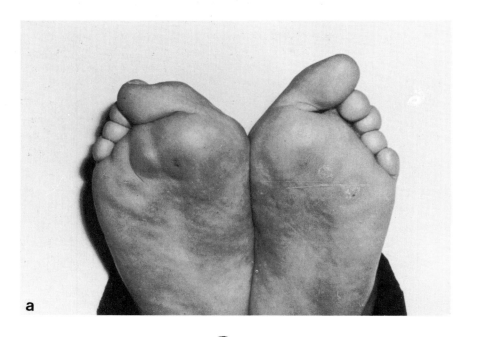

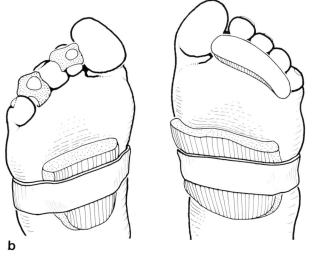

Fig. 4.10. (a) Disabling calosity formation in patient with dropped metatarsal heads resulting from rheumatoid arthritis. (b) Diagram showing pressure relieving pads in place.

AIDS TO MOBILITY

The provision of aids such as walking sticks, crutches, walking frames and wheelchairs is central to the practice of physiotherapy. Precise use of these in the management of patients with rheumatoid disease is important and the guidelines in prescription are the same as for other groups of patients.

There is perhaps one significant difference and that is the emphasis that is given to the consideration of forces or stress put on other joints as a result of using an appliance. For example, in the otherwise healthy orthopaedic patient with lower extremity involvement the stress imposed on the hand, wrist, elbow and shoulder by using crutches is relatively unimportant but in the rheumatoid patient it is significant. It is therefore often necessary to use gutter crutches and modify the handles of standard appliances.

FURTHER READING

AMERICAN ACADEMY OF ORTHOPAEDIC SURGEONS (1975) *Atlas of Orthotics.* C. V. Mosby, St Louis.

MURDOCH G. (1976) *The Advance in Orthotics.* Edward Arnold, London.

5 Hydrotherapy in Rheumatic Conditions

R. A. Harrison

It is generally accepted that hydrotherapy, and in particular pool treatment, has an important part to play in the treatment of rheumatic conditions. It has been estimated [1] that in Britain, at any one time, there will be half a million people with rheumatoid arthritis in need of treatment, and probably there are few of these who would not benefit from the inclusion of some hydrotherapy sessions in their course of treatment.

How many of these patients will receive a planned course of pool treatment will depend upon local circumstances, and regrettably the selection of patients may be reduced to deciding which of those patients will lose least by not receiving it. This makes it imperative that the pool is used to its best advantage and that expensive and valuable facilities are not wasted.

Assessment and planning of treatment

An assessment of the patient is essential to determine the patient's needs, the aims of treatment, and to enable the therapist to decide upon priorities. Every course of hydrotherapy should have a realistic aim, even though it may be necessary to modify this as the treatment proceeds. Assessments are probably best done in the physiotherapy department.

Ideally the patient should be treated by the same therapist for physiotherapy and hydrotherapy but if this is not possible, it is essential that the two therapists should liaise frequently.

Twenty minutes of exercise in warm water is sufficient for the majority of patients if they are not to become uncomfortably hot and overtired. Much can be achieved if this time is well spent and the following points observed:

1. When several joints are involved the therapist must carefully select which joint to treat at any one time, otherwise ineffectual treatment may result because too much is attempted in the short time available.

2. Time should be spent on exercises that can only be effectively carried out in water, and not wasted on exercises that can be done as effectively in the physiotherapy department.

Contraindications

There are no contraindications to pool treatment which are peculiar to the rheumatic diseases, with the possible exception of those patients in the very early stages of recovery from acute generalised episodes of rheumatoid arthritis for whom the treatment with the necessary dressing and undressing may be too tiring. Lists of general contraindications may be found elsewhere [2].

One acute joint need not exclude a rheumatoid patient who would otherwise benefit from pool therapy. The affected joint may be protected from unguarded movements in a purpose-made Plastazote splint.

Abnormal results of physiological measurements (e.g. blood pressure, vital capacity, etc.) should not be total contraindication but rather regarded as warnings. In practice it is only rarely that a patient is excluded from pool therapy for these reasons. If it is thought that a patient would benefit from pool therapy but there is doubt about his suitability, it is better to begin with one or two modified, shorter sessions and assess the effect. Many patients with ankylosing spondylitis, for example, who would have been excluded from pool treatment by too rigid enforcement of the limits of vital capacity often quoted, have received pool treatment and derived benefit.

In those patients with psoriasis the therapist should be aware of, and sympathetic to, the fact that other patients with no knowledge of the disease may be reluctant to bathe in the same water as psoriatic patients. If this situation arises, it will need delicate handling to prevent distress to the patients. Fears can almost invariably be allayed if time is taken to explain the nature of the condition and to point out that the therapists are also in the pool.

When it is essential to keep the hand or foot dry, for example after surgery, a polythene bag can be sealed to the skin with surgical drape. When the upper extremity must be kept out of water a polystyrene raft 50 cm × 50 cm is used.

TREATMENT

The primary aims of treatment are the same for most of the rheumatic diseases:

1. Mobilisation of joints
2. Strengthening of muscles
3. Re-education of function.

Standard hydrotherapy techniques are modified to provide a different approach to various conditions. The approach is determined by whether the condition is acute or chronic, inflammatory or non-inflammatory. Most of the modifications necessary are for the inflammatory joint diseases and in particular for the rheumatoid arthritic patient.

The standard hydrotherapy techniques for strengthening and mobilising are described elsewhere; here only the rationale of the modifications is given with illustrative examples.

Lists of exercises are inappropriate, for the whole concept of treatment is based upon tailoring the treatment programme to fit a particular patient's needs.

Starting positions

Disabled patients often enter the pool from a gantry or hoist and it is natural for the therapist to take them from this to the float lying position. Much of the treatment may then be carried out in this position and they are only transferred to the upright position for formal walking re-education. This is unfortunate because many patients unable to move or stand on dry land find it exhilarating to stand in the pool unaided. For this reason at least part of the exercise scheme should be undertaken in the standing position if possible.

Patients who are nervous of the water are often happier standing and holding the grab rail until they feel more confident. Given a sympathetic and patient approach by the therapist, there are very few patients who do not come to enjoy pool treatments.

Few starting positions are contraindicated, but care must be taken to ensure that in maintaining the starting position strain is not placed on other affected joints.

For this reason, those starting positions which need an overhead grip with the patient in the floating position are contraindicated in most patients with rheumatoid arthritis because of the strain on hands, wrists and shoulders.

Mobilisation

The buoyancy and the warmth of the water promotes general relaxation and specifically relaxation of those muscle groups around painful joints. This is the first step towards mobilisation of these joints.

Mobilisation of joints with contractures must involve stretching of fibrous tissue and because overstretching of periarticular structures may cause a local 'flare-up', the therapist finds herself in a dilemma. In pool therapy this problem is increased by the difficulty of fixation and isolation of a movement to a specific joint. Further the warmth of the treatment pool may encourage the patient to exercise a specific joint too much with consequent adverse effects. It is essential, therefore, that the physiotherapist controls the amount of activity. The experienced therapist is able to judge how much exercise constitutes an optimum treatment session but, until this experience is gained, it is better to 'make haste slowly', always progressing but alert for signs of over-exercise. It is essential to obtain 'feedback' from the patient about the effects of the last treatment and no mobilising treatment should be given before this has been done. After a session of mobilising exercises to a rheumatoid joint one can expect the joint to ache a little for a few hours but certainly after 24 hours this should have subsided. If this is not the case, the next treatment should be modified accordingly.

In a joint which is both stiff and painful, the only way the therapist can be sure that she is having the desired effect is by isolating the movement with adequate fixation.

A scheme of mobilising exercises should, therefore, contain specific exercises of this type as well as more general exercises or activities based on functional patterns. Patients with painful joints may unintentionally perform trick movements to avoid using the painful part; this must be avoided.

Strengthening exercises

Hydrotherapy techniques for strengthening muscles are described elsewhere [2, 3]. All the usual methods of providing resistance to movement in water are used with some small modifications.

In patients with inflammatory joint diseases, it is sometimes difficult to load muscles sufficiently to produce strengthening without at the same time exerting strains on other structures, especially ligaments. One solution is to increase the resistance and adjust the starting position so that the patient works to the maximum but is unable to move the joint and thus performs an isometric contraction. Another possibility is to do the resisted movement in a restricted range choosing that part where the periarticular structures are least vulnerable.

When large floats are used to provide resistance against buoyancy, care must be taken that the patient has control not only of the active strengthening element of the exercise but also of the return movement to the starting position. If this is not done, the patient may lose control of the movement, with possible harmful effects on the joint. This is particularly liable to happen in movements where the effective length of the lever arm increases rapidly towards the end of a movement.

The consequences of using large floats for strengthening should be considered in light of the condition of adjacent joints and the strength of relevant muscle groups.

When floats are used for resistance the therapist should be aware of the amount of resistance they represent, otherwise rational progressions and correlation with treatment in the physiotherapy department cannot be made. All too often physiotherapists use carefully graded weights in the physiotherapy department for the progression of strengthening exercises but when working in the pool use floats with little or no idea of the resistance they are providing. This is unnecessary, for a few simple calculations make it possible to establish the resistance of a particular float or to work out a set of measurements for making a graded series of floats.

A useful basic unit for a set of graded floats is the three inch cube of polystyrene which requires a weight of exactly one pound to submerge it [4].

Swimming

It is common to find patients who, though they can swim, have not done so since the onset of their disease. These patients should be encouraged to swim again and a few minutes at the end of each treatment session devoted to swimming practice. This is usually sufficient for them to gain confidence. In some cases it is worthwhile to allow some treatment time to teach the rudiments of swimming to the non-swimmer.

If the patient can tolerate the temperature of the public swimming baths, a regular visit may have beneficial effects far beyond those of increasing range of movement and strengthening muscles, as it may open up social opportunities. Swimming is an activity in which the rest of the patient's family may participate and it can provide a relatively cheap family outing for those patients whose disability has meant financial difficulty.

More disabled patients may be interested in joining handicapped swimming clubs and the hydrotherapist should be in a position to advise patients on their suitability to do so and of the opportunities which exist locally.

Bad Ragaz

In the past 10 years the type of treatment generally known as the Bad Ragaz Technique has gained increasing importance in the treatment of many conditions. With certain modifications and if care is taken over one or two points, the technique is a useful addition to the treatment regime for rheumatic patients.

An introduction to this technique may be found elsewhere [2, 5, 6] but basically the principles are as follows. The patient performs natural and functional movements usually based upon proprioceptive neuro-muscular facilitation with resistance provided by the forces set up by the movement of the patient's body through the water. Floats are used only for flotation and the counter-pressure for the movement is given by the therapist who is the fixed point about which the patient's movement takes place.

It has been suggested that a minimum pool area of 170 sq. ft is required for Bad Ragaz techniques [6] and in some situations this may rule out its use. Adaptations of the technique for use in a smaller pool have been described [7]. If possible some of these exercises should be incorporated into the scheme not only for their remedial value but because many patients, especially the disabled, enjoy performing these large range, 'free' movements.

In many of these movements the patient moves away from or towards the operator in a free movement which stops only when the limit of the range of movement of the joint is reached, whether this is normal or restricted by contracture. The momentum of the patient often tends to carry the patient beyond this point and whereas in a normal joint this effect is of no consequence, it produces an uncontrolled passive stretching of periarticular structures in a joint with restricted range of movement.

In patients with non-inflammatory joint disease this effect may be used to advantage as a mobilising technique. In those patients with rheumatoid arthritis whose joints are restricted and painful and where uncontrolled stretching is contraindicated, the technique must be modified to prevent this effect which could damage periarticular structures and initiate or increase the inflammatory process.

EXAMPLE 1

The shoulder joint with restricted movement is particularly vulnerable, e.g. in the flexion-abduction lateral rotation pattern. At the beginning of the movement the resistance to the patient provided by the water is great, but towards the end of the movement the patient is moving quickly away from the operator almost feet first with minimal resistance (Fig. 5.1). If the operator were to hold on firmly to the patient's limb when the limit of joint range of movement had been reached, the shoulder joint would be forced into the elevated and abducted position by the patient's momentum. This is obviously undesirable for patients with rheumatoid arthritis or other inflammatory joint disease. The easiest way to obviate this effect is for the therapist to take a short step forward just before the limit is reached and at the same time tell the patient to relax, i.e. to anticipate the next stage of the movement before the limit of range of movement has been reached.

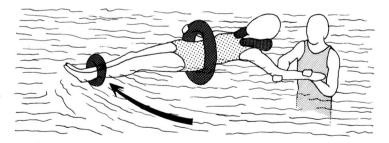

Fig. 5.1. Position of operator to avoid stress on the patient's joint.

EXAMPLE 2

Restricted flexion at the knee joint is often a problem and the single or double knee flexion patterns of Bad Ragaz are useful exercises. Care must be taken, however, when using these exercises that the knee is not forced into uncontrolled flexion. In this movement there is little impedance to the patient's movement through the water (Fig. 5.2) and

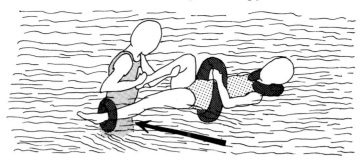

Fig. 5.2. Position for using double knee flexion patterns of Bad Ragaz in patients with painful knee joints.

since the hamstrings are usually strong the patient moves quickly through the water towards the therapist. If the therapist does not allow for this, the knee joints will certainly be pushed forcibly into flexion. This can be prevented, or reduced to an acceptable degree, by modifying the starting position. If the therapist begins the movement with her elbows extended and just before the limit is reached allows her elbows to flex, she will be able to provide the right amount of 'give' necessary to prevent forcible flexion whilst retaining enough of the effect to give a gentle stretching.

Where necessary similar adaptations may easily be made to other Bad Ragaz patterns of movement but they must be practised, preferably on colleagues first, then on patients with non-inflammatory joint disease to get the 'feel' of the technique. This is essential if the therapist hopes to achieve safe controlled stretching using this method of mobilising on patients with rheumatoid arthritis.

The use of the Bad Ragaz techniques for strengthening is straightforward but care must be taken to ensure that in providing sufficient resistance to the muscles one is not inadvertently placing an unacceptable strain on affected joints.

EXAMPLE 3

Lateral strains of the rheumatoid joint inducing stretching of the ligaments may have disastrous effects at a later date. In the double abduction leg patterns where the resistance is given through the lateral side of the foot or ankle a varus strain is put on the knee. In rheumatoid arthritis patients with knee involvement it is better to use single leg patterns with the therapist's hands providing counterpressure and support over the lateral aspects of the knee and ankle joints.

Similar examples will suggest themselves to the therapist.

These exercises can be very tiring for the rheumatoid arthritic patient and it is better to use these techniques interspersed with other exercises which require less effort.

The under current douche

In the spa establishments of Britain many forms of douche were used in the treatment of rheumatic conditions. Most of these are no longer used in National Health Service hospitals. One form however, the under current douche, is still used in some hydrotherapy departments.

The effect is similar to that of the massage manipulation of 'kneading' and is usually directed at muscles rather than joints, being particularly useful for the relief of spasm in the muscles of the neck, back or shoulder girdle.

The under current douche should be regarded as a preparation for treatment by exercise rather than as a treatment in its own right and used in very much the same way as one might use infra-red in the physiotherapy department to promote local relaxation before exercise.

Floats and equipment

Commercially available horse-shoe shaped neck collars are extremely useful. Patients who have specific neck problems may need a Plastazote neck collar to wear beneath their flotation collar, since there is a tendency for the inflatable collar to push the neck into flexion, which even when not harmful may cause discomfort.

Children's inflatable swim-rings and 'trainer' armbands are available in several sizes and a selection of these make a cheap and useful stock of floats for support and resisted exercises. With many disabled patients and those with painful restricted joint movement it may be difficult to manoeuvre them into ring floats and floats of the open sling type are useful. These can be made by enclosing two suitably sized blocks of polystyrene in the ends of a length of stockinette. This type of splint may be slipped under a limb or the trunk and has the advantage that it can be easily adjusted to suit a particular patient.

Much of the pool work with rheumatic patients will necessarily be concerned with the re-education of walking. In some patients there is a discrepancy in leg length and if walking re-education is to be effective, this must be corrected. A heel raise is used, as shown in Fig. 5.3.

Bats are also useful for providing resistance to shoulder movements

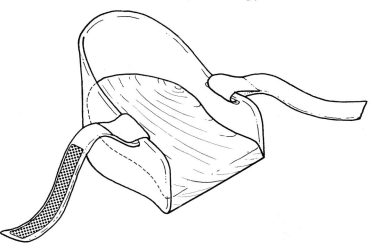

Fig. 5.3. Heel raise used to correct limb length discrepancy in pool.

and if they are used, some should have padded or enlarged handles for patients with restricted finger flexion.

Design and lay-out of pool area

Most therapists will have to use facilities as they exist and this is not the place for a discussion of structural details of a department suitable for the treatment of rheumatic diseases.

There are one or two domestic arrangements, however, which should be made when rheumatic patients are to be treated.

REST AREAS AND PACKING

Most pools will have rest areas attached to them, but if these do not exist, some provision must be made for this type of patient. At its most basic it should consist of a warm well ventilated area where the patient may rest and cool down in a lying position, packed in warm sheets for 20 minutes to half an hour.

LINEN

The requirements for rheumatic patients differ little from those of other patients. A Plombière sheet is particularly suitable for the disabled rheumatic patient. It is simply a large cotton sheet (90 in × 36 in) with an oval hole (8 in × 10 in) at its centre. The Plombière sheet is slipped over the patient's head as he leaves the pool, and has the double advantage of permitting easy removal of a wet bathing suit and of keeping the patient warm.

ATTENDANTS

Physiotherapy aides, bath hall attendants and porters are required to lift and handle patients in the pool area. Their general training should include instruction in the lifting of patients. The handling of rheumatoid patients has special dangers and it is the responsibility of the physiotherapist to ensure that all personnel understand how to lift such patients without discomfort or injury to painful joints and to avoid injury to those with 'tissue paper' skin.

The effective treatment by hydrotherapy of patients with rheumatoid disease has improved considerably in recent years with a more reasoned approach. It is essential that hydrotherapy techniques for the treatment of rheumatoid arthritis are constantly evaluated and modified in response to the ever increasing knowledge about the medical and physiotherapy management of this group of patients.

REFERENCES
[1] MASON M. (1977) *Rheumatism – The Price We Pay*. The British League against Rheumatism, London.
[2] BOLTON E. & GOODWIN D. (1974) *An Introduction to Pool Exercises*. Churchill Livingstone, London.
[3] DUFFIELD M. H. (ed.) (1976) *Exercises in Water*. Bailliere Tindall, London.
[4] HARRISON R. A. (1980) A quantitative approach to resisted exercise in pool treatment. *Physiotherapy*, **66(2),** 60.
[5] DAVIS B. C. (1967) A technique of re-education in the treatment pool. *Physiotherapy*, **53(2),** 57.
[6] DAVIS B. C. (1971) A technique of resistive exercise in the treatment pool. *Physiotherapy*, **57(10),** 480.
[7] BOLTON E. (1971) A technique of resistive exercise adapted to a small pool. *Physiotherapy*, **57(10),** 481.

6 Rheumatoid Arthritis

Rheumatoid arthritis is the most common connective tissue disease and certainly the most important in socio-economic terms; it has been estimated that 37 million working days per annum are lost as a result of rheumatoid disease. The predilection of the disease for females, in a ratio 3:1, has a far reaching effect on family life and in any treatment programme this factor must be considered.

The prescription of appropriate physiotherapy in rheumatoid disease is determined by physical assessment of the patient and consideration of what is known of the disease process, its aetiology, pathogenesis and clinical features. Detailed accounts of the latter are abundant in the literature and should be reviewed for specific information. Here it is pertinent to highlight salient points with regard to the natural history of the disease and the clinical features it manifests, since these are essential in determining patient care.

AETIOLOGY

This remains unknown. Speculative theories suggest that immunological and genetic factors may play a role in the disease and much research has concentrated on identification of an infective agent, but to date more is known about the pathogenesis of the disease than its cause.

PATHOLOGY

Principal pathological changes occur in the synovium, in the arteries and in the formation of subcutaneous nodules but, as discussion of the clinical features will show, manifestations of the disease are widespread.

SYNOVIUM

Initially this becomes thickened, oedematous and congested and then proliferates and hypertrophies until there is formation of profuse granulation tissue, which invades the articular cartilage, and forms the characteristic pannus. The synovial pannus breaches the cartilage eroding into subchondral bone, and once this has happened the combined effect of mechanical forces and continued inflammatory process leads to erosion of bone and ultimately joint destruction.

It is important to note that the synovial changes can occur in all synovium so the linings of tendons and bursae are also affected.

ARTERIES

Arteritis may occur in:

1. Small end arteries – more commonly seen in the digital vessels around the nail bed.
2. Small arteries, resulting in skin ulceration.
3. Large arterial vessels, leading to gangrene.

SUBCUTANEOUS NODULES

These are characteristic, occurring in 25% of patients with rheumatoid arthritis. A common site is the ulnar border of the forearm (Fig. 6.1).

Stages of the disease

It is usual to describe the progression of the disease in three stages:

Stage I   Synovium only involved
Stage II   Early articular cartilage involvement
Stage III Destruction of joint surfaces.

CLINICAL FEATURES

Onset of the disease may be at any age, although commonly it begins in the fourth decade. This systemic disease may exhibit a wide spectrum of

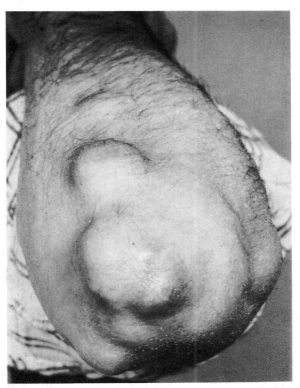

Fig. 6.1. Subcutaneous nodules on forearm in patient with rheumatoid arthritis.

symptoms, but at onset it usually presents as an inflammatory arthropathy of the sero-positive group and may be polyarticular, monoarticular or palindromic. The course of the disease is erratic and unpredictable.

Symptoms

Pain and stiffness are predominant. Initially pain may only occur with movement but as the disease progresses is present at rest. Morning stiffness is so characteristic that it is often used as an index of the disease.

Pattern of joint involvement

Typically the metacarpophalangeal joints are first affected followed by involvement of the proximal interphalangeal, wrist, metatarsophalangeal, knee, shoulder and hip joints. Cervical spine involvement may also occur early in the disease [1].

ARTICULAR SIGNS

SYNOVIAL HYPERTROPHY

This is typically doughy on palpation and distinctive from the effusion found in a joint following trauma. Early in the disease it may be seen as fusiform swelling in the proximal interphalangeal joints giving rise to the characteristic spindle shaped fingers (Fig. 6.2).

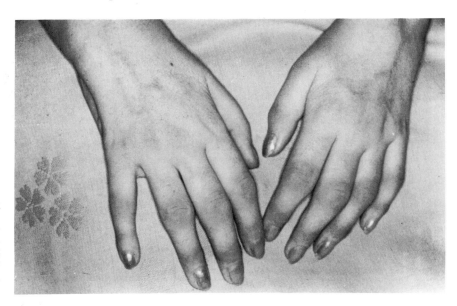

Fig. 6.2. Typical fusiform swelling of interphalangeal joints in early rheumatoid arthritis. Note swelling over metacarpophalangeal joints.

SUBLUXATION AND JOINT INSTABILITY (Fig. 6.3)

These are seen later in the disease and are due to persistent stretching of the joint capsule and ligaments causing laxity of these structures.

PRESENCE OF CHARACTERISTIC DEFORMITY

Deformity occurs in late stages of the disease and results from a combination of the altered joint architecture due to erosive changes and

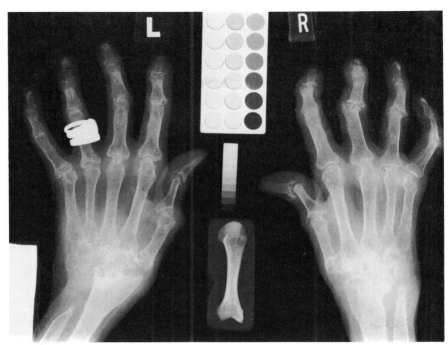

Fig. 6.3. Radiograph of hands in late stage rheumatoid arthritis. Note gross erosions of carpus.

disturbed mechanics; the product of changes in the dynamic functions of tendons, muscles and ligaments.

In the hand. Ulnar deviation (Fig. 6.4) at the metacarpophalangeal joints.

Swan neck deformity of the fingers (Fig. 6.5) – this arises from hyper-extension of the proximal interphalangeal joint with fixed flexion of the terminal interphalangeal joint.

Boutonnière deformity (Fig. 6.6) – the proximal interphalangeal joint protrudes through the extensor expansion, the two halves of which slip forward until attempts to extend the joint produce flexion at this joint but extension at the terminal interphalangeal joint (Fig. 6.7).

In the wrist. Early erosive changes in the ulnar styloid and, later, cystic changes in the distal ends of both radius and ulna, lead to a position of palmar flexion and deviation.

In the feet. Subluxation of the metatarsophalangeal joints, with the toes displaced upwards and fixed flexion at the interphalangeal joint, results in dropped metatarsal heads. These then become weight bearing.

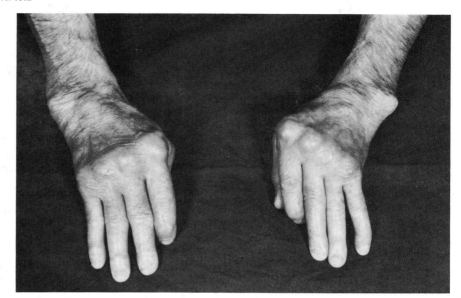

Fig. 6.4. Ulnar deviation in patient with rheumatoid arthritis.

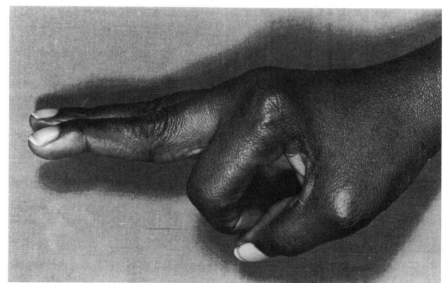

Fig. 6.5. Swan neck deformity.

In the cervical spine. The involvement of the cervical spine occurs early in the disease, as neither the synovium surrounding the odontoid peg nor the transverse ligament of the atlas are spared. The problem is not so much one of deformity but of instability, with subluxation at the atlanto-axial joint (Fig. 6.8).

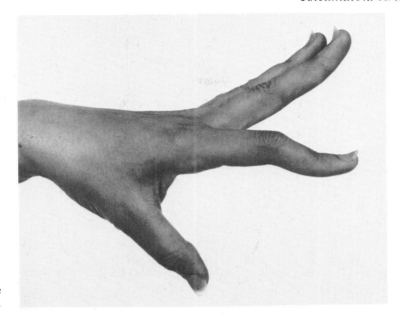

Fig. 6.6. Boutonnière deformity.

SWAN NECK DEFORMITY

Intrinsic imbalance "spasm" →
1. Increased flexion pull at MCPs
2. Increased extension pull at PIP and DIP → hyperextension at PIP joint

BOUTONNIÈRE

Weakening of central slip of extensor tendon, change of function of lateral bands of tendon →
1. Constant flexion pull at PIP
2. Hyperextension at DIP

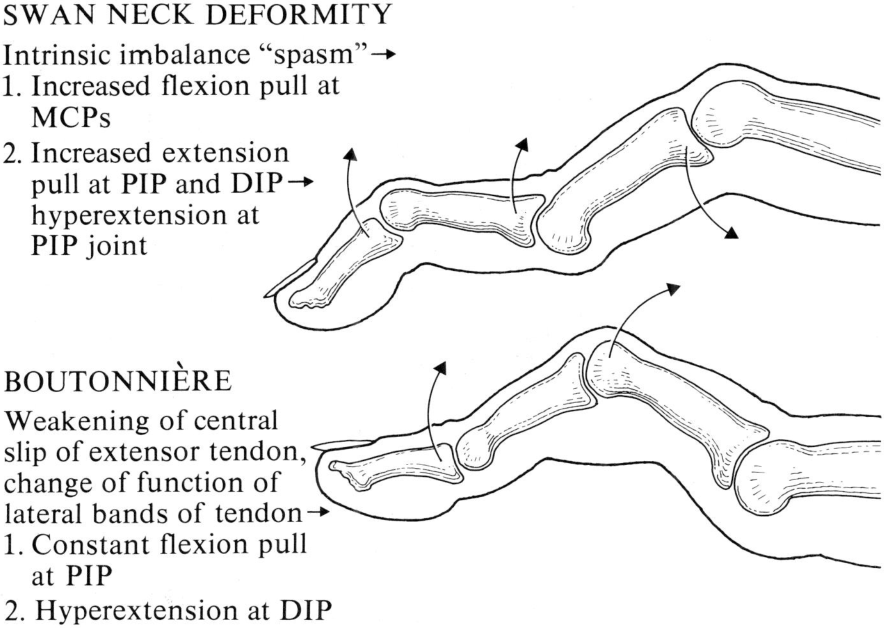

Fig. 6.7. Diagram to show mechanism of swan neck deformity and boutonnière deformity.

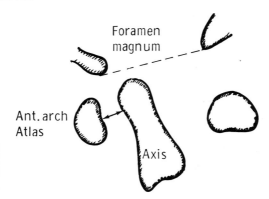

Fig. 6.8. Schematic representation of atlanto-axial subluxation.

In the hips. Flexion deformity with external rotation occurs. The hip joint may also be compromised by aseptic necrosis of the femoral head, which is seen as a complication of corticosteroid therapy (Fig. 6.9).

In the knees. Flexion deformity with varus or valgus components.

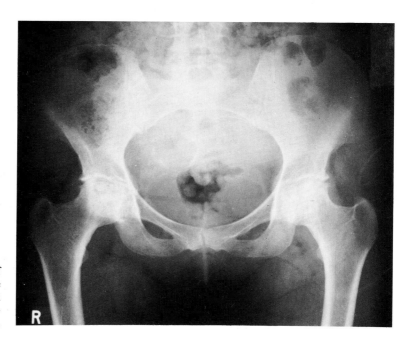

Fig. 6.9. Radiograph of left hip showing collapse of the femoral head from aseptic necrosis, steroid-induced.

EXTRA-ARTICULAR SIGNS

   1. Fever and weight loss
   2. Lymph node enlargement
   3. Subcutaneous nodules
*4. Involvement of tendons and bursae
   5. Arteries
*6. Spinal cord compression
*7. Peripheral neuropathy
*8. Lungs and pleura
   9. Skin
 10. Anaemia
*11. Myopathy

*Those extra-articular features of rheumatoid disease that are amenable to treatment by physiotherapy are asterisked and discussed in more detail in the following paragraphs.

TENDONS

The normal function of tendons may be impaired by synovitis and/or thickening of the tendon sheath. Teno-synovitis gives rise to minor swellings palpable along the course of the tendon which may only produce slight discomfort, and may resolve spontaneously.

Direct invasion of the tendon by granulation tissue may also occur, the tendon becomes frayed and elongated and eventually may rupture (Fig. 6.10). The long flexors, extensors and extensor pollicis are more frequently involved.

Tendons are the link by which the contractile force of muscle is transmitted to bony levers; any change in tendon length or integrity results in altered mechanics, both dynamic and static. The hand and wrist are particularly vulnerable to these changes and it has been estimated that in more than 50% of patients presenting with rheumatoid disease tendon involvement is seen [2, 3].

The wrist joint is a common site for rupture of the extensor tendons. This results from a combination of wrist flexion deformity causing an imbalance of long extensors, long flexors and intrinsics. In the advanced disease where distal radio-ulnar dislocation occurs, the dorsally displaced ulna may be an additional factor in causing rupture of the extensor tendons.

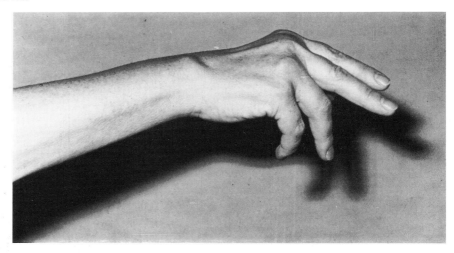

Fig. 6.10. Hand of patient with rupture of the extensor tendon to ring and small finger.

Involvement of the long extensor at the level of the metacarpophalangeal joint results in anterior subluxation. The normal movements at the metacarpophalangeal joint are limited by the collateral ligaments and the hood mechanism of the extensor expansion.

Attenuation and stretching of the middle slip insertion of the extensor aponeurosis at the proximal interphalangeal joint results in flexion of the joint with extension occurring at the distal interphalangeal joint.

SPINAL CORD COMPRESSION

The spinal cord may be compressed at the atlanto-axial joint where subluxation occurs or at the base of the skull with erosion of the odontoid peg. It has been demonstrated that there is considerable disparity between the radiological incidence of cervical spine subluxation and the incidence of clinical manifestation of cord compression (Fig. 6.11a, b).

Signs of upper motor neurone involvement may appear gradually and are often masked by the gross muscle weakness and pain-induced muscle spasm of the systemic disease. The physiotherapist should be alert for early signs of upper motor neurone lesion in treating rheumatoid patients and, in those patients with known cervical spine involvement, must use care in selecting treatment positions that do not jeopardise the upper cervical spine. In clinical practice it is our observation that increased tone in the calf muscles is one of the early positive signs identified.

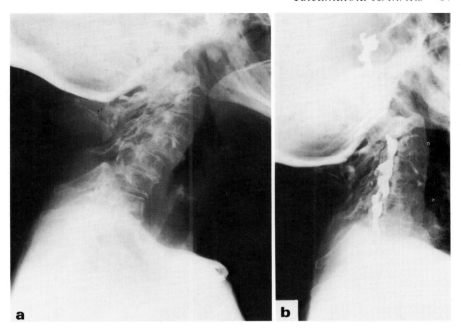

Fig. 6.11. (a) Radiograph of the cervical spine in a patient with advanced rheumatoid arthritis. (b) Same patient one year later.

PERIPHERAL NEUROPATHY

Entrapment neuropathy. The most common lesion is one of compression of the median nerve at the wrist giving rise to the carpal tunnel syndrome. According to one study [4] it is seen in up to 50% of cases of early rheumatoid arthritis. Other entrapment neuropathies are seen, but less frequently, for example the ulnar nerve at the elbow.

Neuropathy of vascular origin. Symmetrical peripheral neuropathy may be a distal sensory neuropathy or a sensorimotor neuropathy (Fig. 6.12). Mononeuritis multiplex is rare and is the result of ischaemic interruption of peripheral nerves.

LUNGS AND PLEURA

Rheumatoid disease may manifest itself in the lungs as:

1. Pleural effusions
2. Acute diffuse interstitial fibrosis
3. Chronic diffuse interstitial fibrosis
4. Rheumatoid pneumoconiosis
5. Lung nodules

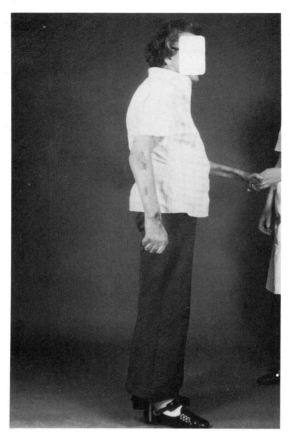

Fig. 6.12. Patient (Mrs J. – see case history) walking with below knee caliper. Note gross wasting of the upper extremities from neuropathy.

The incidence of lung involvement is reported to be small but this may be an under-estimation. The patient may remain asymptomatic but with radiological changes in the lungs evident. The use of steroids in the management of the systemic disease may also be responsible for masking early symptoms.

MYOPATHY

The muscular atrophy which occurs is profound and integral to loss of functional capacity. The cause of the atrophy is not clearly understood, it was originally thought to result from the cycle of pain, loss of mobility, protective muscle spasm, pain that leads to disuse atrophy. It has been demonstrated on muscle biopsy [5] that in mild rheumatoid arthritis patients there is atrophy of Type II fibres, while in severe rheumatoid there is atrophy of Type II fibres with selective involvement of Type I fibres. In a similar study [6] differential changes in Type I and Type II fibres were found and it was postulated that in some cases of rheumatoid arthritis there is a very early involvement of muscle, with atrophy that is not simply of disuse.

It would seem then that the atrophy may be caused by:

1. Pain and immobility – producing disuse atrophy
2. Reflex inhibition of muscle, caused by pain
3. Reflex inhibition by mechanoreceptors acting over distended joints
4. Possible direct involvement of muscle
5. Secondary steroid-induced myopathy

Diagnosis

Diagnosis is quite apparently not the province of the physiotherapist but an understanding of some of the diagnostic tests and their significance is important. Interpretation of the tests is fundamental to designing appropriate treatment programmes.

CLINICAL TESTS

Erythrocyte sedimentation rate
Anaemia
Urine
Rh. factor
Salicylate levels

See Appendix A.

Features of rheumatoid arthritis seen on radiological review are:
Presence of erosions
Presence of soft tissue calcification
Changes in joint space
Osteoporosis
Subluxation of joints

TREATMENT

The management of the patient with rheumatoid arthritis is most effective where a team approach is used and it is usual for the following disciplines to be included by the rheumatologist:

1. Medical social worker
2. Occupational therapist
3. Orthotist
4. Physiotherapist
5. Nurse

Additionally the orthopaedic surgeon, plastic surgeon and disablement rehabilitation officer have important roles at specific times in the patient's management.

General guidelines

Although the number of joints and the extent to which they are involved at any stage of the disease will vary, it is essential that the patient as a whole is treated. The level of disease activity is not constant for all joints at the same time.

Drugs

Analgesics
Anti-inflammatory drugs
Steroids
Gold
Penicillamine
For the effects and side effects of these drugs see Appendix 'B'.

Rest

General. Rheumatoid disease has widespread systemic manifestations and these, combined with significant and often unremitting pain, make rest essential for the patient. The term rest requires some clarification because in common usage it can mean taking to one's bed. The patient therefore needs to be carefully counselled that 'rest' means taking adequate time between activities to avoid fatigue. The balance between activity and rest is determined by the level of disease activity.
Local. Opinion varies regarding the effect of imposed rest by immobilisation on peripheral joints, although it is now generally accepted that judicious immobilisation is beneficial and with care does not in-

crease joint immobility. The period and degree of immobilisation appears to depend on the rheumatologist's opinion, gained from experience.

In this unit complete immobilisation of peripheral joints is not used and we rely on rest splints with or without the use of isometric exercises. However, other groups of workers [7, 8] report beneficial effects from immobilisation of patients with Stage I, II and III rheumatoid disease.

Most patients with rheumatoid disease are managed on an out-patient basis.

Role of the physiotherapist in the out-patient rheumatology clinic

A physiotherapist attends out-patient clinics to:

1. Assess and re-assess patients
2. Communicate patient's progress
3. Offer advice on the indication for physiotherapy and the most appropriate form of treatment
4. Review and revise home programmes
5. Review and adjust, as necessary, splints and appliances

Out-patient department attendance is only indicated where:

1. The patient has just been diagnosed as having rheumatoid arthritis
2. There has been rapid or marked deterioration
3. There is a specific aim and objective of treatment

There are still those patients for whom hospitalisation is thought to be beneficial. Criteria for admission vary but in this unit are:

1. Early diagnosis – stabilisation of drug therapy
2. Where there are multitudinous and complex problems to be reviewed, or where the patient's condition has deteriorated rapidly
3. Social reasons

In other units the need for intensive rehabilitation might be an additional criterion.

PHYSIOTHERAPY

Aims

1. To educate the patient
2. To maintain and restore muscle power

3. To maintain and restore joint range and patient mobility
4. To prevent deformity
5. To correct deformity
6. To maintain optimum function and physical performance
7. To relieve pain

Methods

EXAMINATION AND ASSESSMENT

The first step in good management is examination and assessment; only after this has been thoroughly undertaken can the specific aims of treatment for the individual be defined and the programme outlined.

Since the disease is rarely static, frequent re-assessment is necessary, both to monitor the effect of therapy and to redefine treatment goals.

Details of methods of examination and assessment are found in Chapter 3.

PATIENT EDUCATION

From the first contact with the patient the physiotherapist should involve the patient and his/her relatives in the treatment, explaining carefully the purpose of exercise and rest and the balance between them.

The patient is taught how to protect vulnerable joints from further damage and the importance of good posture and body mechanics at work and leisure is emphasised.

Where there is loss of function the physiotherapist helps the patient to find alternative ways of accomplishing the activity. It is in this respect that the physiotherapist needs to familiarise herself with the patient's home and work environment. The extent to which the physiotherapist is involved in ergonomics and the provision of aids and adaptations in the home depends on the practice of a particular rheumatology unit. Ideally the occupational therapist undertakes much of the functional retraining but it is essential that close co-operation exists between the two disciplines.

A list of local and national voluntary services that may be contacted for advice should be available to the patient.

Maintenance and restoration of muscle power

The long course of the disease and the primary or secondary effect that it has on muscle makes it essential for the patient to perform strengthening exercises daily.

The scheme of exercises given to a patient is designed for his particular needs and is routinely revised to take account of improvement or progression of the disease. This revision has the further effect of motivating and encouraging the patient.

Progressive resisted exercises are most effective, but where these are used careful supervision is essential, at least in the first few weeks, to ensure that the resistance is not increased at the expense of range or stress on joints and that the patient fully understands that exercise must be within the limit of pain. It is not sufficient to simply tell the patient to exercise within pain tolerance, the instruction must be specific, that is, if increased pain is felt and lasts for more than two hours after exercise then the amount of exercise should be curtailed and only built up again slowly. Such instruction will avoid increasing the irritability of joints and enhance the chances of the patient's compliance with a home routine.

Resisted mat work is used to re-educate the use of the postural reflex mechanisms (Fig. 6.13).

Proprioceptive neuromuscular facilitation is particularly helpful in strengthening the muscles of the extremities and trunk stabilisers (Fig. 6.14). Techniques of repeated contractions, slow reversals and rhythmic stabilisations are those of choice. Where there is pain and joint instability considerable skill is needed, quick stretch and approximation

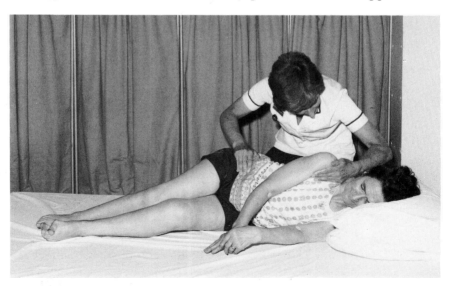

Fig. 6.13. Mat work – resisted rolling.

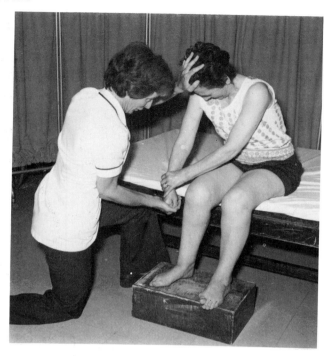

Fig. 6.14. Trunk flexion. Note modified position of leading hand.

should be avoided and the rotation components of movement must be carefully controlled (Fig. 6.15).

Resisted walking techniques (Fig. 6.16) are helpful in strengthening the muscles acting over the hip, knee, ankle and foot. Approximation through the hips can be used judiciously, but where pain in the hip, knee or ankle joint is marked the pelvis is guided forward and joint compression avoided.

In emphasising the use of maximum resistance as a method of strengthening, it must be stated clearly that maximum resistance is that amount that can be overcome by a smooth co-ordinated contraction throughout range. In the rheumatoid arthritic patient failure to observe this dictum means an increase in joint swelling, pain and deleterious strain on already impaired joint structures.

Maintenance and restoration of joint range and patient mobility

Maintenance. Normal daily activity, particularly where this is limited by pain and disability, does not maintain full range of movement. Patients are encouraged to put joints through full range movements daily;

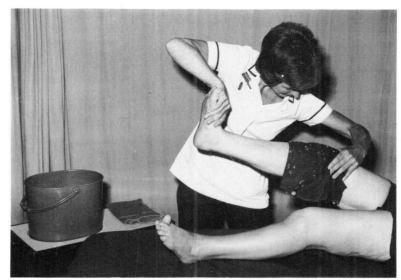

Fig. 6.15. Repeated contractions inner range knee extension in flexion adduction, external rotation with knee extension.

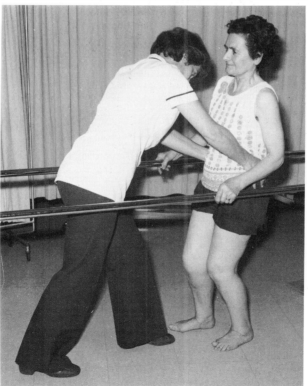

Fig. 6.16. Resisted walking.

active movement is preferred but it is sometimes necessary to use active assisted movement. Passive movement is not indicated. Patients are cautioned about accepting insidious limitation and advised to establish objectives.

Restoration of range. Repeated active movements into the limited range are encouraged and should be performed several times per day. Soft tissue limitation may be amenable to passive stretching, accomplished by using the force of gravity, e.g. in obtaining hip and knee extension by prone lying or by teaching the patient or a relative to gently use sustained pressure on tight structures.

The physiotherapist uses techniques of hold relax, contract relax and repeated contractions to gain range of motion.

Hydrotherapy is also beneficial in restoration of joint range (see Chapter 5).

It cannot be over-emphasised that range of motion without voluntary control is of doubtful value and, in patients with rheumatoid disease where joint instability is often a problem, may even be detrimental.

The use of splints to gain range of motion is discussed later in this Chapter (p. 79).

Mobility. Methods of re-education of walking have already been discussed (p. 74). In the patient with rheumatoid disease the importance of independent ambulation must be carefully considered in relation to stress imposed on other joints and energy cost.

Prevention of deformity

Characteristic deformity develops in rheumatoid arthritis as the disease progresses. Initially the patient tends to habitually adopt joint postures that afford most relief of pain, usually ones that reduce tension over the swollen joint capsule and its irritable synovial lining. Secondary to this, there is lengthening of the ligamentous structures on one side of the joint and contracture or shortening on the other. Inevitably, muscle atrophy with resultant muscle imbalance, together with pain-induced muscle spasm, contribute to this process, particularly in those postural muscles whose function it is to maintain the body in the erect position, namely quadriceps femoris and glutei.

In the advanced stages of the disease destruction of bone by erosion causes deformity as the bony contours are no longer able to glide smoothly over opposing surfaces. In the weight bearing joints the process is hastened by the abnormal stresses produced during attempts to walk with changed and even bizarre gait patterns, resulting from altered body mechanics.

Utmost vigilance by the physiotherapist is mandatory if deformity is to be prevented, for it is apparent that changes occurring in one joint, once measurable, must already have imposed abnormal postures and strain on the joints above and below. For example, a 10° knee flexion contracture will almost certainly have already limited the degree of hip extension the patient uses in normal walking, therefore the cadence is changed and the weight acceptance of both hip joint and ankle altered. The methods used in preventing deformity are:

1. Patient education
2. Exercise
3. Passive stretching
4. Splintage

Careful explanation to the patient about the dangers of adopting poor postural habits is essential. The patient should be counselled not to use pillows under the knees at night and to avoid undue stress on the wrists both in work and in activities of daily living, for example using the hands to push up the body weight when rising from a chair. The patient is advised on postural correction exercises and is made aware of the importance of correct posture.

Exercise to maintain muscle strength and range as previously described is important in preventing deformity.

The patient is carefully instructed in the correct method of passively stretching joint structures (*not* passive movements) and when the patient is unable to perform this herself, a relative is instructed. It is not sufficient merely to tell the patient how to passively stretch the joint, it must be carefully demonstrated and then supervised until the physiotherapist is confident that the correct method is firmly established. When this is not done, over stretching may occur and other deformities provoked.

REST SPLINTS

These are used judiciously in the prevention of deformity, particularly in the hand, wrist and knees. They are indicated when the joint is acute, that is the disease process is active, the joint being swollen and painful with muscle spasm present. The splint is made to encourage relaxation and should not attempt over-correction. It is important that the splint is well lined to avoid any chafing or pressure points and it must also be easy for the patient to apply (see p. 32).

Rest splints are usually necessary only at night but in very acute joints or where the patient is immobilised for any reason it many be necessary that they be worn for periods during the day.

The patient is instructed that if the splint is uncomfortable after wearing for several hours, it should be removed and the skin inspected and a note made of any areas of redness. Those patients who find it difficult to tolerate splints are advised to wear the splint for only one or two hours at a time, until they have become accustomed to them.

Whenever a physiotherapist makes splints for a patient she should ensure that the patient is seen for review within a week, preferably the next day. Unfortunately all too often patients give up wearing splints, because they are uncomfortable, and develop a negative attitude to any external device, although a minor adjustment to the splint could make it acceptable to them.

WORKING SPLINTS

These are used (a) where joints are at risk from stress, and (b) to improve function. Work splints are commonly used for the wrist. A variety of splints or orthoses to protect the weight bearing knee and ankle joints are available. For details of these see p. 37.

Correction of deformity

If deformity does occur there is no indication for correction unless it will improve function and/or relieve pain.

Correction may be achieved by:

1. Conservative methods
2. Surgical intervention (Chapter 7)

Where there are several joints with fixed deformity, the order in which correction is attempted must be carefully considered by evaluating the effect that correction will have on the joint above and below.

CONSERVATIVE METHODS

1. Serial splinting
2. Intensive muscle strengthening programme
3. Skin traction

Before embarking on serial splinting it is essential to ensure radiologically that there is sufficient joint space left to permit correction and to establish the degree of osteoporosis. A description of serial plasters is found on page 34.

Intensive strengthening exercises are undertaken simultaneously and increased range of motion is not sought until the patient has voluntary control over the existing range. Accurate measurements of joint range and muscle power are made at frequent intervals.

The use of skin traction for correction of deformity in the lower extremity of adults was discontinued in this unit because it was found to have a limited effect, which did not outweigh the disadvantage of confining the patient to bed and the possible development of skin lesions. However, in the management of children with rheumatoid disease the method has more merit (see Chapter 8).

Maintenance of function and physical performance

Pain and loss of muscle power and mobility are all too frequently the hallmarks of rheumatoid arthritis but it may be argued that it is loss of functional capacity that causes the most physical and emotional distress to the patient. Unfortunately, disturbance of function and the significance of this to any individual patient cannot be correlated with joint involvement or stages of the disease. For example a young housewife with Stage I rheumatoid arthritis may suffer more disturbance of function than a patient with obvious deformity of Stage III rheumatoid arthritis.

Specific, controlled and localised physiotherapy may improve function by increasing muscle power, joint range and mobility. The ultimate objective of any rehabilitation programme is to improve function and this requires close co-operation with the occupational therapist. The physiotherapist in designing the exercise programme must reinforce patterns of movement taught by the occupational therapist to achieve the patient's personal care, activities of daily living and work requirements.

The importance of rest in the acute phase of the disease, when exercise has to be kept within the limit of pain and fatigue if deleterious effects are to be avoided, has already been discussed. However, there is evidence to suggest that in the non-acute stage a programme to enhance physical performance is indicated and improves function. Studies undertaken in Sweden [13, 14, 15] showed improvement in physical performance and function in the test group of 34 patients with Stage II or III rheumatoid arthritis following a period of physical training. The joint status of the patients remained unchanged. A similar study [16] also demonstrated improvements using a training programme that patients undertook at home. Further, a small increase in muscle fibre size was found and a correlation between muscle strength and Type II fibre size.

The vicious cycle of muscle atrophy of disuse, incapacity and poor physical performance may be broken by giving patients a home programme of physical training.

Relief of pain

Historically many rheumatoid patients have been referred for physiotherapy with the primary objective of pain relief. Heat has been administered by various methods: hot packs, short wave diathermy, infrared and paraffin wax baths. There is as yet little objective evaluation of these methods and no evidence to support the view that they have any effect on the underlying pathology. However, there is no doubt that, clinically, patients often report that previously stiff joints 'feel looser'. This subjective finding is probably the result of relaxation of muscle spasm and therefore the use of these modalities as an adjunct to exercise may be justified. As research and evaluation of physiotherapy techniques develop, evidence to support other claims for these methods of treatment may be found.

Cooling muscle and skin to temperatures low enough to affect the conduction velocity of nerve is most efficacious in reducing muscle spasm and in relieving pain [12]. The most effective method is application of ice towels which are changed frequently.

Perhaps the most important point to remember is that pain is the body's natural defence mechanism and the physiotherapist exercising a joint following prolonged cooling must use caution and skill and not abuse a joint made vulnerable.

If the patient is admitted to hospital for treatment, in addition to the methods previously described a ward class is helpful (Fig. 6.17).

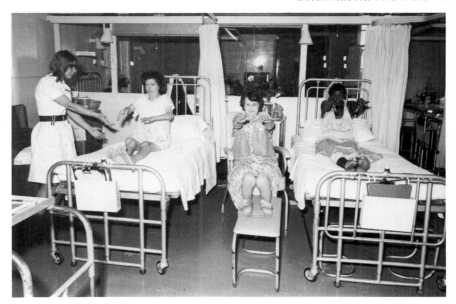

Fig. 6.17. Ward class.

The ward class has the advantage of:

1. Teaching and instilling in the patient the value of daily exercise.
2. Providing an opportunity for patient education.
3. Group support.

The short and long term effects of hospitalisation on patients' functional and social status and the influence on prognosis are a subject of concern and have been studied in depth [9, 10, 11].

Lastly, regardless of whether the patient has required in-patient treatment or has had a course of out-patient treatment, a home programme is essential.

A home programme is determined by the examination and is specific for each patient. Emphasis may be on lower trunk, hip and knee extensors or muscle groups of the upper extremity. *Isometric exercises* using a near maximum contraction are very useful, particularly where pain is significant. It is of utmost importance that the programme is reviewed and altered to meet the patient's changing need. The frequency of the review will depend on the level of disease activity.

Community care

The role of the community physiotherapist in the management of rheumatoid arthritic patients is similar to that of other patients with long term chronic disease and the provision of services is documented [17].

Case history

Mrs J. Age 59 years. (See Table 6.1 and Fig. 6.18.)
January 1973
Onset of pain in right wrist, shoulders, metacarpophalangeal joints and knees. Erythrocyte sedimentation rate raised.
   Diagnosis: Sero positive rheumatoid arthritis.
   Drugs: Phenylbutazone, indocid, and gold with good response.
September 1973
Gold stopped because of albuminuria.
December 1973
Developed mononeuritis multiplex involving lateral popliteal and ulnar nerves.
   Drugs: Penicillamine and systemic steroids.
June 1974
   Drugs: Penicillamine stopped, chlorambucil started.
July 1974
Admitted to Hammersmith Hospital.
   Findings: Symmetrical distal sensorimotor neuropathy, marked muscle weakness, bilateral claw hands with flexor tendon contractures, dropped feet, sacral pressure sores. Totally dependent, could not do anything for herself. Unable to walk for past 2–3 months.

Table 6.1. Quantitative assessment of patient (Mrs J.) with rheumatoid arthritis and vasculitis.

Date	21.8.75		18.9.75	
	Right	Left	Right	Left
Function				
Grip strength (mmHg)	134	75	139	94
Walking time (sec) (30 yards)	45 (with frame)		39 (unaided)	
Muscle strength (Newtons × 10)				
Shoulder abduction	9	8	9.5	9.5
Wrist extension	10	7	11.5	8.5
Hip flexion	10	10	12.0	9.5
Hip extension	8	6	8.0	8.5
Knee extension	10	8	15.0	12.5
Knee flexion	4	3	4.5	2.5

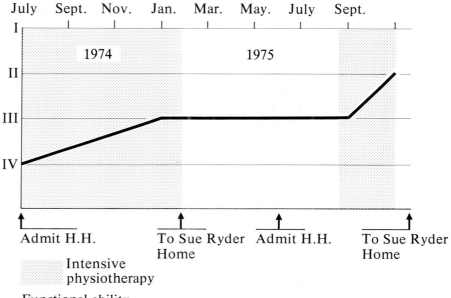

Fig. 6.18. Graph showing functional ability of patient related to periods of intensive physiotherapy.

Functional ability

I   Totally independent
II Minimal help
III More help
IV Totally dependent

Muscle biopsy: Left vastus lateralis Type II fibre dystrophy.

Drug therapy: Chlorambucil stopped. Systemic steroids raised to 60 mg then slowly reduced.

Physiotherapy: Ward class – active free exercise, manually resisted exercises to strengthen, functional rehabilitation, lively splints for hands.
January 1975
Discharged to Sue Ryder Home. Steroids 25 mg/day. Fully mobile walking with Zimmer frame. Minimal change in hands – persistent flexor contractures.
May 1975
Developed indolent leg ulcers. Re-admitted. Phenol lumbar blocks performed.
August 1975
Transferred to Rheumatology unit for intensive rehabilitation.

Findings: Marked distal neuropathy both hands and feet. Claw hands with flexion contractures (Fig. 6.19), no activity right intrinsics, slight

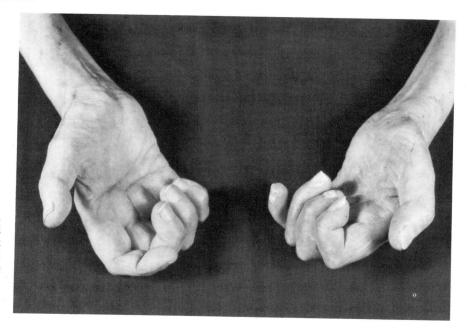

Fig. 6.19. Flexion deformity of PIP and DIP joints in a patient with rheumatoid arthritis, note atrophic changes in skin and nail. Patient is attempting to extend fingers.

activity left intrinsics and left hypothenar muscles. Both hands very painful and sensitive to touch. Cannot manage Zimmer frame but can walk with considerable support. Wears light drop foot calipers. Ulcers on lower legs healing but requiring daily dressing.

Physiotherapy: Ward class – free active exercise. Manually resisted exercises to strengthen especially trunk, and lower and upper limbs. Facilitating with strong neck musculature and bilateral limb patterns. Stretch plasters and massage and stretching four times daily for hands. Massage for leg ulcers. Functional rehabilitation.

October 1975

Full extension of fingers following serial stretch plasters; these were used because it was felt that the deformity was the result of tendon tightness. Hands free of pain. Independent in self care, mainly because of increased hand function. Walking independently but uses rollator for long distances. Ulcers healed.

November 1975

Returned to Sue Ryder Home. Probable final diagnosis: rheumatoid arthritis vasculitis with distal sensory motor neuropathy with attempts at treatment resulting in steroid myopathy.

REFERENCES

[1] FLEMING A., CROWN J. M. & CORBETT M. (1976) Incidence of joint involvement in early rheumatoid arthritis. *Rheumatology and Rehabilitation*, **15**, 92–96.

[2] BREWERTON D. A. (1957) Hand deformities in rheumatoid disease. *Annals of the Rheumatic Diseases*, **16**, 183–197.

[3] BREWERTON D. A. (1969) Radiographic studies of tendons in the rheumatoid hand. *British Journal of Radiology*, **42**, 487–492.

[4] BARNES C. G. & CURREY H. L. F. (1967) Carpal tunnel syndrome in rheumatoid arthritis. A clinical and electrodiagnostic survey. *Annals of the Rheumatic Diseases*, **26**, 226–233.

[5] BROOKE M. H. & KAPLAN H. (1972) Muscle pathology in rheumatoid arthritis, polymyalgia rheumatica and polymyositis. *Archives of Pathology*, **94**, 101–118.

[6] EDSTRÖM L. & NORDEMAR R. (1974) Differential changes in Type I and Type II muscle fibres in rheumatoid arthritis. *Scandinavian Journal of Rheumatology*, **3**, 155–160.

[7] GAULT S. J. & SPYKER J. M. (1969) Beneficial effect of immobilisation of joints in rheumatoid and related arthritides: A splint study using sequential analysis. *Arthritis and Rheumatism*, **12**, 34–44.

[8] PARTRIDGE R. E. H. & DUTHIE J. J. R. (1963) Controlled trials of the effect of complete immobilisation of the joints in rheumatoid arthritis. *Annals of the Rheumatic Diseases*, **22**, 91–99.

[9] DUTHIE J. J. R., BROWN P. E., KNOX J. D. E. & THOMPSON M. (1957) Course and prognosis in rheumatoid arthritis. *Annals of the Rheumatic Diseases*, **16**, 411–424.

[10] DUTHIE J. J. R., BROWN P. E., TRUELOVE L. H., BARAGAR F. D. & LAWRIE A. J. (1964) Course and prognosis in rheumatoid arthritis. A further report. *Annals of the Rheumatic Diseases*, **23**, 193–202.

[11] CONATY J. P. & NICKEL V. L. (1971) Functional incapacitation in rheumatoid arthritis: a rehabilitation challenge. *Journal of Bone and Joint Surgery*, **53A**, 624–637.

[12] LEE J. M., WARREN M. P. & MASON S. M. (1978) Effects of ice on nerve conduction velocity. *Physiotherapy*, **64(1)**, 2–6.

[13] EKBLOM B., LÖVGREN O., ALDERIN M., FRIDSTROM M. & SÄTTERSTRÖM G. (1974) Physical performance in patients with rheumatoid arthritis. *Scandinavian Journal of Rheumatology*, **3**, 121–125.

[14] EKBLOM B. *et al.* (1975) Effect of short-term training on patients with rheumatoid arthritis I. *Scandinavian Journal of Rheumatology*, **4**, 80–86.

[15] EKBLOM B. *et al.* (1975) Effect of short-term physical training on patients with rheumatoid arthritis – a six month follow up study. *Scandinavian Journal of Rheumatology*, **4**, 87–91.

[16] NORDEMAR R., BERG U., EKBLOM B. & EDSTRÖM L. (1976) Changes in muscle fibre size and physical performance in patients with rheumatoid arthritis after 7 months' physical training. *Scandinavian Journal of Rheumatology*, **5**, 233–238.

[17] PARTRIDGE C. J. & WARREN M. D. (1977) *Physiotherapy in the Community*. Campfield Press.

7 Surgical Management of Rheumatoid Arthritis

Surgical intervention is indicated at different stages of rheumatoid arthritis but the decision to proceed with surgery is complicated by the erratic and often unpredictable nature of the disease and by the fact that commonly many joints, tendons and ligaments are affected by the disease process. When surgery is undertaken there is always a specific aim for the procedure.

Indications for surgery may be summarised as:

1. Relief of incapacitating pain
2. Restoration of stability
3. Improvement in function
4. Prevention of harmful stresses on other joints

It is of paramount importance that before any procedure is decided upon a full assessment of the patient is made by all members of the team including the physiotherapist. The careful examination of joint range, muscle power and function (Chapter 3), when reviewed, will help the surgeon to determine the procedure and the likelihood of a successful outcome and will reveal the patient's major problems when several joints are involved.

In a patient with only one badly affected joint, for example the hip, the decision is relatively simple, but in a patient with gross bilateral involvement of joints in both upper and lower extremities the decision is complex. Major surgery of the lower extremity with the period of non-weight bearing, when crutches must be used, may provoke further exacerbation of pain and deterioration in the hands and elbows. During the period of assessment and pre-operative treatment the physiotherapist is able to gauge the patient's motivation and likely compliance with postoperative rehabilitation regimes.

Surgery in rheumatoid joints basically consists of three types of procedure:

1. Synovectomy
2. Arthroplasty
   a. Excision
   b. Interposition
   c. Partial joint replacement
   d. Total joint replacement
3. Arthrodesis

The type of procedure chosen will depend on the stage of the disease, that is whether the disease process has involved articular surfaces as well as synovium, the joint involved and the number of joints.

The normal function of tendons and ligaments is frequently affected in the rheumatoid patient, resulting in pain, instability of joints and malfunction. The surgeon operates to perform reconstruction, repair and tenolysis on the affected tendons.

There are inevitably so many surgical procedures, each with various modifications, that no attempt is made in the following paragraphs to discuss these in detail but only to outline general principles.

SYNOVECTOMY

In Stage I rheumatoid arthritis where only the synovium is affected and there are no apparent changes in the geometry of the joint synovectomy is the procedure of choice. Synovectomy is usually performed only on the knee, metacarpophalangeal, wrist and elbow joints. The rationale of the procedure is evident; by removing the diseased synovium it is hoped to retard the progression of articular destruction and prevent further synovitis. A controlled trial [1] has shown that pain, synovitis and joint destruction may be delayed for at least three years by early synovectomy.

The knee

PREOPERATIVE PHYSIOTHERAPY

This consists of:

1. Breathing exercises

2. Intensive quadriceps strengthening exercises
3. Intensive hip strengthening exercises in particular for the hip extensors and abductors
4. General mobilising and strengthening exercises for all other joints
5. Posture correction
6. Instruction in the use of crutches, either axillary, elbow or gutter depending upon the degree of involvement of upper extremity joints.

POSTOPERATIVE PHYSIOTHERAPY

The speed with which the postoperative physiotherapy programme is advanced will depend on two factors: the individual surgeon's preference for early activity and the response of the patient, which should be constantly monitored. A basic programme is as follows:

Days 1–10
Breathing exercises
Intensive isometric quadriceps exercises
Intensive hip extension and abduction exercise
Participation in the ward class for general mobilising exercises

Periods of lying supine and, if there is any suggestion of hip flexion tightness, lying prone. By strategically placing pillows, pressure is avoided over the incision, which will in any case be protected by a large pressure bandage.

Depending upon skin healing, which is often slower in rheumatoid patients, alternate stitches are usually removed around the tenth day. At this stage some surgeons permit gentle knee flexion exercises, others prefer to wait up to three weeks. Whenever knee flexion exercises are started two important points must not be overlooked:

1. The patient must always be able to achieve full extension actively;
2. Any sign of increased pain or swelling means that the exercise has been too rigorous.

The most useful techniques in gaining flexion are hold relax and contract relax; ice towels over the whole bulk of the quadriceps muscle are a helpful adjunct.

Partial weight bearing is usually commenced during the third week and the knee is supported by a posterior plaster of Paris slab. This will continue to be worn until the patient has at least 60° of controlled knee flexion.

If improvement in range of knee flexion reaches a plateau before the patient has obtained a useful range, i.e. 100°, the surgeon may wish to manipulate the knee under general anaesthesia. When this is done, ideally the physiotherapist should be in theatre to observe (a) the degree of force needed and (b) the range gained. Immediately the patient is fully conscious, the physiotherapist starts encouraging the patient to actively obtain the range gained. Ice towels placed over the knee joint and bulk of the quadriceps will relieve pain and facilitate relaxation of the quadriceps. It is of paramount importance that strong quadriceps exercises are given at the same time, so that a quadriceps lag is not permitted to develop. The patient is seen for short treatments at least four times a day during the following week.

The wrist and shoulder

Synovectomy at the wrist and shoulder is rarely done as an isolated procedure (see page 96).

The elbow

Synovectomy at the elbow is considered a useful procedure. Gentle free active exercises are usually commenced 3–4 days postoperatively. The patient is encouraged to move the elbow through flexion and extension for short periods several times a day. Pronation and supination of the forearm should also be encouraged. Once the patient has obtained full range of motion, further physiotherapy is not indicated. Attention to shoulder and hand movements is necessary until the patient is using the arm normally.

ARTHROPLASTY

Excision arthroplasty

In this procedure peri-articular bone is resected and the space so formed becomes filled with scar tissue during the healing process. The effect is to create a mobile, painless but unstable joint, the instability occurring because the joint capsule and ligaments are no longer under tension. In the major weight bearing joints such as the hip and knee the inherent instability is so detrimental to function that the operation is rarely used, except as a salvage procedure, and in the knee is always accompanied by another procedure, e.g. arthrodesis.

THE FOOT

In the foot excision arthroplasty is of great benefit, often completely relieving the patient of the persistent and disabling metatarsalgia that results from the subluxation of the metatarsophalangeal joints. There are two procedures commonly used, Fowler's and Keller's operations. *Fowler's procedure* involves excision of the metatarsal head and proximal part of the proximal phalanges. *Keller's operation* consists of removal of exostosis from the medial aspect of the first metatarsal and excision of the proximal third proximal phalanx of the great toe.

Physiotherapy

Little specific physiotherapy is necessary postoperatively for these patients although it is a useful precaution to review the gait pattern and of course ensure that maintenance exercises are performed during the ten days that the patient is relatively immobile. Some surgeons wish their patients to have a short course of faradic foot baths and intrinsic foot exercises commencing one month after surgery. The physiotherapist is well advised to look at the patient's footwear, since in most cases the shoes used preoperatively will no longer be suitable.

THE ELBOW

Here the commonest procedure is excision of the radial head with or without synovectomy. This leaves the patient with a fairly stable joint that is painfree. However, it is only of value when the changes are confined to the lateral compartment of the joint.

Although procedures involving excision of part of the humeral condyles are described, it is of doubtful merit in the severely involved rheumatoid because the joint will certainly be unstable and prohibit the use of walking aids.

Postoperative physiotherapy

Simple exercises to maintain range of elbow flexion and extension are given, together with pronation and supination exercises. There is rarely need for more than a few days of treatment. It is essential to monitor the patient's hand function and grip strength.

Interposition arthroplasty

In this procedure debridement of the joint is performed and a foreign material is interposed between the joint surfaces. The material may be either Silastic® or metal and covers only one joint surface; for example, a vitallium cup lining the acetabular portion of the hip joint articulates with the femoral head.

THE HIP

This type of arthroplasty in the hip is performed less commonly now in rheumatoid patients because it requires a longer period of non-weight bearing and hospitalisation. Total hip replacement is now the procedure of choice.

THE SHOULDER

Anatomical features of the shoulder joint have made this joint less amenable to successful joint replacement than the knee or hip. The peculiar problems are the enormous range of motion that this joint permits and the shape of the articular surfaces, for example the size of the humeral head in relation to the glenoid cavity. Stability of this joint is entirely due to the effect of the stabilisers, supraspinatus, subscapularis, infraspinatus and teres minor.

An endoprosthesis is used to replace the humeral component and the muscles of the rotator cuff are repaired. Physiotherapy commences at the end of the first week with very gentle pendular exercises and does not progress until after three weeks when the surgeon may permit more active work.

Patients who have undergone arthroplasty of the shoulder need a long period of rehabilitation.

Techniques of proprioceptive neuromuscular facilitation are particularly useful and patterns utilising the neck and scapular are used to enhance the effectiveness of the scapular and shoulder muscle stabilisers. Attention is necessary to ensure that a reversed scapulo-humeral pattern is not developed.

THE KNEE

In this joint various prosthetic devices are used, sometimes involving one or both tibial plateaus and more rarely the condylar part of the femur. Physiotherapy is similar to that for total knee replacement.

Total joint replacement

THE HIP

This is the most frequently replaced joint and although there are innumerable prostheses and modifications used, they all have common features of a femoral component fitted into the medullary canal, often cemented into place, and an acetabular portion which is cemented into the acetabulum (Fig. 7.1).

The type of prosthesis is unimportant to the physiotherapist but postoperative physiotherapy is influenced by the structures cut during surgery. For example some surgeons resect the greater trochanter and then wire it back, which obviously compromises the muscles attached, namely gluteus medius. As always, it is essential to read the operation notes before proceeding with physiotherapy.

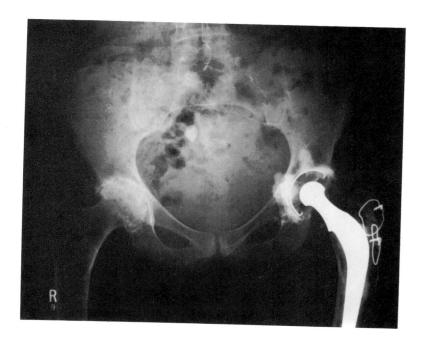

Fig. 7.1. Radiograph showing Charnley total left hip replacement with wiring of greater trochanter. Note loss of joint space of right hip.

Postoperative physiotherapy

The patient is returned from theatre with a drain *in situ*. A wedge is placed between the thighs to prevent adduction and internal rotation as this is the position in which the hip is unstable and the possibility of dislocation exists. The patient is nursed flat.

1–3 days. Breathing exercises
   Isometric gluteal contractions $\big\}$ the affected leg
   Isometric quadriceps exercises
   Isotonic quadriceps exercises – for the unaffected leg
   Foot and ankle exercises
   General maintenance for the upper extremities and trunk
   Postural correction
   *SLR should *not* be done

3–10 days. Exercises continue as above. Patient is allowed up weight bearing using two sticks. The emphasis is on walking re-education because the patient who has walked with considerable pain for many months/years prior to surgery will inevitably have developed a poor gait.

   Care is needed in getting the patient up as sitting is not permitted, that is flexing the hip to 90° is avoided, until 6 days, although gentle small range hip and knee flexion exercises are given. At this stage internal and external rotation exercises are commenced.

10–14 days. The physiotherapy programme outlined is advanced to include stronger exercises. The patient is full-weight bearing, if the other joints permit.

14–21 days. The patient is discharged home. The physiotherapist checks that the patient is able to perform all activities of daily living.

   Out-patient treatment is rarely necessary.

THE KNEE

Total knee replacement (Fig. 7.2) has developed more slowly than total hip replacement, primarily because of the difficulties of developing an artificial joint that could withstand the rotational forces acting over the joint.

   As with the hip there are several varieties of prosthesis available but they may be grouped into four basic types.

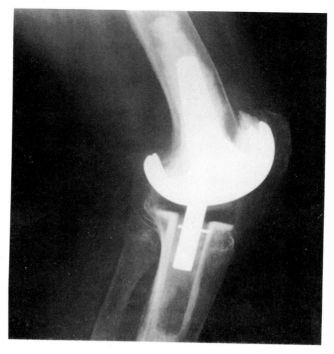

Fig. 7.2. Radiograph showing Attenborough prosthesis *in situ* left knee.

1. The simple hinge permitting only flexion and extension.
2. Devices that replace both condyles and the midline tissues and although not linked by an axle, as in the hinge joint, are linked to prevent some of the abduction adduction and rotation occurring at the knee.
3. Devices that replace the whole knee but are not linked.
4. Devices that replace the condyles only.

Preoperative physiotherapy

Breathing exercises
Intensive quadriceps strengthening
Intensive hip extension exercises
General mobility exercises.

Postoperative physiotherapy

Orthopaedic surgeons differ enormously in their preference for early mobilisation of patients following total knee replacement. In some units the patient is mobilised within 48 hours and discharged home within a week, whilst in other units vigorous mobilisation does not commence before three weeks. Nevertheless, the aims of physiotherapy are the same, strengthening of the quadriceps muscles and knee flexors and restoration of range of motion. It is essential that the patient is not permitted to develop a quadriceps lag because this will make the knee inherently unstable and therefore emphasis is given to working the inner range of the quadriceps muscle.

Attention should also be given to the hip extensors and abductors, as these will often be weak.

In contrast to the patient with total hip replacement these patients often require a short period of out-patient physiotherapy.

ARTHRODESIS

Where arthrodesis is performed in the major joints, the physiotherapy is as for arthrodesis performed for any orthopaedic condition. It is in reaching the decision to proceed with fusion that the physiotherapist has a role to play. Since the altered mechanics and increased forces subsequently placed on the adjacent joints of the rheumatoid patient are significant, the physiotherapist's assessment must explore the detrimental effects and the implications for self care activities.

Cervical fusion

Physiotherapy after cervical fusion in the rheumatoid patient is essentially the same as when this procedure is undertaken for other reasons. However, meticulous care to prevent deformity and painful stress on other joints during the postoperative period is essential. Since in many cases the disease will have already caused profound muscle atrophy, particular attention to general muscle strengthening is mandatory.

The indications for chest physiotherapy will depend on the incision and approach used, e.g. where a trans-oral approach is used, tracheostomy is performed.

SURGERY OF THE HAND IN RHEUMATOID ARTHRITIS

The normal hand is a complex instrument used both for fine precision work and for powerful movements, it is required to be stable and yet capable of extremes of dexterity. These almost diametrically opposed objectives are achieved by a composite of bony articulations, architecturally so well conceived, and a system of levers and pulleys so delicately balanced that execution of the most skilled movements is possible. To use the modern idiom the packaging of this tool is so remarkably accomplished that the hand is relatively small and is aesthetically pleasing. It is not surprising therefore that even minor insults to the joints, tendons or muscles cause disturbance of function and in rheumatoid arthritis the disruption of tendons and muscles with impending destruction of articular surfaces is often devastating.

The inter-relationship between muscle, tendon, capsule, ligaments and joint in the hand is so close that for clarity the surgical procedures are described for each joint.

The wrist

Synovectomy of this joint as an isolated procedure has already been mentioned but more commonly it is seen in association with tendon repair and/or excision. Rheumatoid disease may compromise the radiocarpal, the inter-carpal or inferior radio-ulnar joints and the tendons of the extensor or flexor compartments. In the early stages of disease the patient may only present with synovitis of the ulnar and radial bursae with locking or hitching of the flexor tendons; a tenosynovectomy is then performed. In more advanced stages, the disease may cause subluxation of the carpus anteriorly, destruction of the inferior radio-ulnar joint and dorsal protrusion of the remaining ulnar stylus with possible laceration of the extensor tendons. Any encroachment of the wrist produces impairment of hand function with reduction in grip power. Reconstructive surgery is performed as early as possible and may involve a combination of synovectomy of the wrist, excision of the inferior radio-ulnar joint, repair of tendons and synovectomy of the extensor compartment.

Physiotherapy is directed toward restoring joint range and hand function. If the tendons have been repaired movement is usually delayed until the third week but where these have not been sutured, wrist movement is commenced at one week. Ice and techniques of repeated contractions using the shoulder and elbow for reinforcement and overflow are particularly helpful. Serial measurements of grip strength are used to monitor progress.

Arthrodesis of the wrist joint is indicated in some patients and when this is undertaken the position of fusion is carefully determined. It is often helpful to stabilise the wrist with a temporary splint and re-measure grip strength and re-assess function to demonstrate improvement before proceeding with surgery. If only unilateral arthrodesis is considered, the position is usually one of 15°–25° extension but where both wrists are fused one should be in a neutral or slightly flexed attitude so that the patient's self care ability is not affected.

The metacarpophalangeal joints

These joints are notoriously involved and as the disease progresses, swelling, instability, ulnar drift, contracture of the intrinsics, palmar subluxation and palmar dislocation of the proximal phalanx may all be seen. The mechanism by which these occur and the rationale of surgical intervention is more easily understood by reference to the anatomical arrangement. The metacarpophalangeal joint is a gliding joint and does not have a fixed centre for rotation. It relies for stability on the balance between the extensor expansion of extensor digitorum and the intrinsic muscles, the strong collateral ligaments, and the capsule which is separate. The direction of the ligaments is such that the joint is stable in flexion, but when in extension, the movements of abduction, adduction and rotation are permitted.

As the extensor tendon and ligaments are invaded by the disease ulnar drift starts to occur, the extensor expansion sliding towards the ulnar side of the joint with attenuated or ruptured radial collateral ligaments. This may be compounded by tightness or contracture of the intrinsic muscles, which are normally active in flexion, and palmar subluxation with anterior dislocation of the proximal phalanx occurs.

Simple synovectomy of the joint with intrinsic release and re-alignment of the extensor mechanism suffices to restore function where dislocation has not yet occurred and the ligaments and articular surfaces are relatively intact, but with more advanced disease arthroplasty or joint replacement is indicated (Fig. 7.3). As in other regions of the body there are many varieties of prosthesis available, the most frequently used are the Swanson, Calnan-Nicolle and Flatt prostheses.

POSTOPERATIVE PHYSIOTHERAPY

Physiotherapy commences:
  After synovectomy in 2–3 days

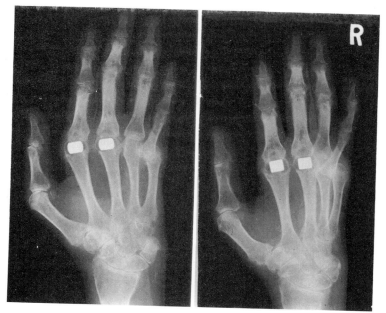

Fig. 7.3. Radiograph showing prosthetic replacement of 2nd and 3rd metacarpophalangeal joints.

After synovectomy with collateral ligament repair or extensor re-alignment in 5–7 days

After arthroplasty in 10–14 days

After prosthetic replacement in 2–3 days where dynamic splints are used [2], in 2–3 weeks where dynamic splintage is not used and a volar support is preferred. At three weeks a dynamic splint is then fitted and further physiotherapy as an out-patient is usually unnecessary.

The general aims of physiotherapy are to restore the movement of flexion and extension and improve hand grip and function by increasing muscle strength. Where intrinsic release has been performed, care must be taken to prevent hyperextension deformity at the proximal interphalangeal joint and the extensor digitorum sublimus must be particularly strengthened. After synovectomy and arthroplasty there is some risk of lateral instability, therefore abduction and adduction movements should be avoided or limited.

Proximal interphalangeal joints

In health these joints move only in a single plane but in rheumatoid disease they are subject to deforming forces as the tendons and ligaments are weakened.

The classical boutonnière deformity occurs when the flexor digitorum pulls unopposed by the tendinous insertion of extensor digitorum, which becomes thinned and weakened, and the finger is held in flexion.

Limitation of flexion at the interphalangeal joint is seen in the swan neck deformity which occurs when the extensor digitorum and intrinsics become tight and dorsally displace the lateral bands.

These joints are similarly managed surgically with synovectomy, repair and prosthetic replacement.

Carpometacarpal joint of thumb

This is a fundamentally unstable joint relying on muscle and ligamentous attachments rather than on bony configuration. In advanced rheumatoid disease this joint is prone to dislocation and contracture of the capsule producing an adducted thumb.

Surgery at this joint is usually removal of the trapezium with resiting of the abductor pollicis longus more distally. Sometimes a Silastic spacer replacement is inserted.

The MCP joint of the thumb

The typical deformity at this joint is one of flexion and it gradually occurs as the dorsal hood becomes distended and weakened and the extensor pollicis longus tendon becomes displaced in an ulnar direction until it finally lies below the rotational axis of the joint. Any attempt to actively extend the joint then produces flexion.

The integrity and stability of the MCP joint is vital for pinch grip, loss of weakness of pinch grip being a severe functional impairment.

Fusion of this joint is the most satisfactory procedure.

REFERENCES

[1] ARTHRITIS AND RHEUMATISM COUNCIL AND BRITISH ORTHOPAEDIC ASSOCIATION (1976) Controlled trial of synovectomy of knee and metacarpophalangeal joints in rheumatoid arthritis. *Annals of the Rheumatic Diseases*, **35**, 437–442.

[2] NICOLLE F. V. & PRESSWELL D. R. (1975) A valuable splint for the rheumatoid hand. *The Hand*, **7**, 67–69.

8 The Management of Arthritis in Children

R. E. Jarvis

Arthritis in children may present at any age and in a variety of ways. Early diagnosis of juvenile arthritis enables treatment to be started before severe deformities occur rendering the child chairbound and incapable of leading an independent life. The overall prognosis is considerably better than in adult rheumatoid disease, but there are different types of disease patterns and while remissions occur in some patients, others may continue with relapses for many years, with resulting radiological changes.

The different types of the disease can be described as follows:

Systemic disease

In the younger age group, namely one to five years of age, systemic disease is common, often with the involvement of multiple joints. These children can be very sick with a high swinging fever, maculopapular rash, enlarged lymph nodes, hepatosplenomegaly, and in some cases pericarditis.

Pauci-articular

In contrast to the systemically ill child, this group may appear reasonably fit with up to four joints involved. They may have the added complication of iridocyclitis, which can lead to blindness if not treated.

Polyarticular disease

There are many joints involved in this type of disease and although the child may not be systemically ill, there may be constitutional features present, for example anaemia, which will make the child listless and appear generally unwell.

Juvenile rheumatoid arthritis

This is usually found in the older age group of children with onset around puberty; girls are more frequently affected than boys. It is a more aggressive form of arthritis with muscle weakness and joint deformities occurring very early in the course of the disease. The small joints of the hands and feet are commonly affected, as in the adult rheumatoid patient, and there are also features of the disease seen in the younger age group.

Juvenile ankylosing spondylitic group

These patients often present with peripheral joint involvement, for example ankle or knee, and eventually go on to develop ankylosing spondylitis. Boys are more frequently affected than girls and onset is usually around the age of puberty.

Other conditions

Arthritis can be associated with a number of other conditions, for example psoriasis, in which there is asymmetrical joint involvement and, if not managed correctly, severe loss of function.

GENERAL MANAGEMENT

The management of these children is a complex one, involving a team of people including doctors, nurses, physiotherapists, occupational therapists, medical social workers, chiropodists, teachers, parents and friends. Communication among all these people and with the child is essential to ensure that maximum benefit is obtained from treatment, and throughout the child's school and social activities.

To control the disease activity and enable the patient to become as fit as possible an anti-inflammatory analgesic drug regime is necessary. Should the disease activity continue over a long period, drugs aimed at reducing the overall rheumatic activity need to be considered. Corticosteroid therapy may be used.

PHYSICAL MANAGEMENT

The physical management of all types of juvenile arthritis is basically the same. The patient requires constant observation for the correction of poor habits and immediate treatment of any joint which is showing signs of disease activity. In the initial stages of treatment considerable patience and understanding by the therapist are necessary to gain the confidence of both the child and his parents, thus ensuring co-operation from all concerned in the child's welfare. The problems are numerous and whereas the younger ones seem able to come to terms with the disease, the teenagers are much more difficult to manage because in addition they have the problems of adolescence. A basic regime of exercises, suitable splinting, prone-lying and adequate rest combined with schooling and social activities is necessary to overcome the mental and physical problems, and enable the child to grow up to become a contributing adult in the community.

Aims of physiotherapy

1. To maintain and improve muscle function and power
2. To maintain and improve joint mobility and function
3. To prevent deformity
4. To rehabilitate the patient to become independent and lead a normal life as far as is possible

The most common joints to be affected are the neck, wrists, hands, knees and ankles. Hip involvement is seen in about 40% of cases and usually develops after prolonged activity of the disease. The physiotherapist must be vigilant for other joint involvement and treat as necessary; for example, the temporomandibular joint may become insidiously stiff and daily exercise to this joint should therefore be included in the basic scheme of exercises.

It must be remembered that arthritis is a painful condition and a child in pain is unwilling to move and will take up the position of most comfort, usually flexion. The child is often miserable and introverted and requires confidence to realise that he can lead a relatively normal life if he can learn to manage his own body and cope with the pain and stiffness. Independence in all activities is the keynote to success. In some patients it is complete independence, in others varying degrees of independence. Movement to stimulate growth and prevent osteoporosis is essential in the child. The rate of growth in a normal person is rapid, but with prolonged disease activity, juvenile arthritis may slightly retard growth.

Exercises

The active child does not put his joints and muscles through a full range of movements during normal everyday activities; therefore, a scheme of basic exercises for each muscle group and joint must be carried out daily and be continued for many years, even when the disease appears quiescent, as joints will stiffen and fuse if not kept mobile (Fig. 8.1).

In the more painful stages of the disease, these exercises must be performed twice daily. The movements should be active on the part of the child or active assisted with the help of the therapist or parent. The child should be encouraged to move the joint to the limit of his pain tolerance, then return it to the starting position, following this with the same movement again, trying to take it a little further each time. By this method the child will gain confidence in his own ability to improve the range of movement by gradually increasing the muscle power and overcoming the pain barrier (Fig. 8.2).

In the systemically ill child, position in bed is most important, with the knees and ankles supported in back slabs to prevent flexion con-

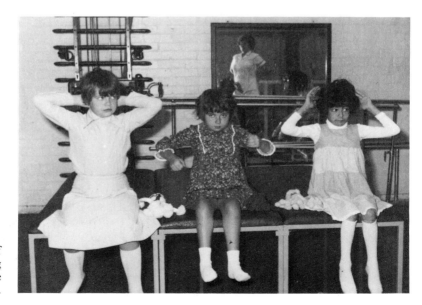

Fig. 8.1. Group of patients performing general exercise programme.

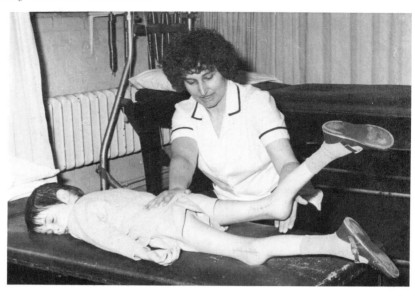

Fig. 8.2. Patient with hip and knee flexion contractures receiving assistance and encouragement from physiotherapist.

tracture of the hips and knees and foot drop. The wrists and hands should also be supported in splints to keep the wrists in a good functional position. During this phase it is most important that exercises are carried out twice daily. Active assisted movements of all muscle groups are necessary to keep the joints mobile and as the child improves he must be encouraged to become more active. The length of time taken to remobilise him varies with each individual and relapses may occur at any time.

Back extension exercises are of paramount importance to prevent the round shouldered appearance so often seen in the patient with arthritis. The ability to move the scapula round the chest wall is lost in some children and an extension movement of the spine is produced with the shoulders held forward. In this case the child needs assistance to make sure that the exercise is performed correctly (Fig. 8.3).

Breathing exercises are important for all cases of juvenile arthritis, in particular for those with the ankylosing type of the disease, as the expansion of the chest wall tends to become limited in a very short time.

Quadriceps and gluteal exercises need special attention so that walking with hips and knees flexed is avoided. Springs and slings can be used to add resistance to these muscle groups and also assist movement of the hip and knee joints.

Ankle and foot movements are necessary if the child is to maintain

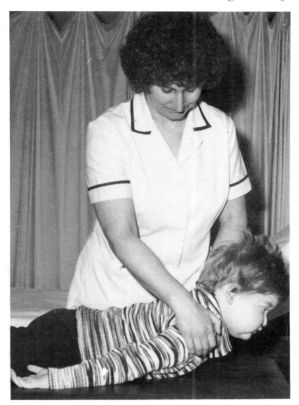

Fig. 8.3. Back extension exercises. Note the cushinoid appearance from corticosteroid therapy.

the correct pattern of walking and balance. Eversion of the foot is often the most difficult movement for the patient to perform, therefore exercises to strengthen the evertor muscles should be shown to the child and the parent. The metatarsal area of the foot can also present a problem and movement of the metatarsals can help in relieving the pain and enable the child to walk using the whole of his foot.

Shoulder movements are often difficult and exercises to the shoulder joint are made easier if performed in the lying position so that gravity is eliminated. Full elevation of the shoulder may require some assistance from the therapist or parent until the child is able to perform the movement himself. Elevation through both flexion and abduction with lateral rotation is performed, taking care that a reversed scapulo-humeral movement is not taught.

Basically, flexion and extension of the elbow joint is a simple movement; however, to obtain a greater range of extension, the child may perform the movement with the forearm in pronation. If this is not corrected so that the extension of the elbow is carried out with the forearm in supination, loss of extension and supination results.

Extension of the wrist is necessary to enable the fingers to function properly. All movements should be carried out with the emphasis on strengthening the wrist extensor muscles. Individual exercises to each joint in the fingers will keep the tendons free and grip strengthening exercises should be given. Opening a door is one of the most important everyday activities that the arthritic child must perform.

The neck can present a problem and extension is one of the movements which becomes very limited. Active exercise in all directions is important and posture correction of the neck may be necessary. The parent may need considerable guidance with this, as limitation of extension and a torticollis are often not noticed by a person close to the child.

Hydrotherapy

Water is an ideal medium for the treatment of children with arthritis. The heat relieves the pain while the buoyancy assists the movement of the limbs. Both individual and group activities can be carried out in a hydrotherapy pool and a play session for the younger age group can be included as this is a medium in which physical handicap is at a minimum. Swimming, as the sport of choice at any age, should be encouraged to allow the competitive spirit of the child to develop.

The use of the hydrotherapy pool for the treatment of the lower limbs is most important. Hip and knee movements can be encouraged without putting undue strain on the joints and walking re-education can be started in the pool in preparation for mobilisation on dry land (Fig. 8.4).

The two to ten year old child, once confident in the pool environment, responds well to treatment in the water. The very stiff knee can often be mobilised subconsciously by the child if his mind is on other activities, for example, playing with a friend or learning to swim.

The bath is an ideal substitute for the hydrotherapy pool, but does limit the movements of the hips. However, for the patient at home, a daily bath, in which most of the exercises can be carried out, greatly assists him in overcoming early morning stiffness. The child under the age of two is happier if treated in a bath than in an enormous pool. He may also be incontinent.

Independence in dressing and undressing can be learnt at this time, with periods of training in using aids, if necessary.

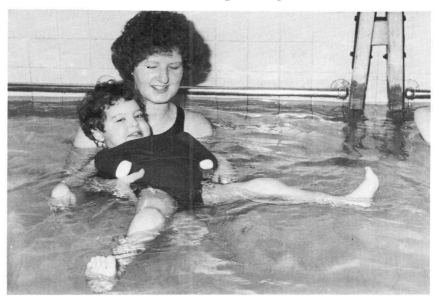

Fig. 8.4. A three year old using the water to assist hip movements.

Prone-lying

Prone-lying plays an important role in the management of this disease. A period of rest in prone-lying is advisable for at least one hour a day in order to keep the hips and back extended. In hospital, prone-lying can be carried out after lunch, by lying across the bed or with the feet over the end of the bed to allow the ankles to rest at right angles to the leg and prevent plantar flexion of the ankle and internal rotation of the hips. In the case of the child at home, it is advisable for him to prone-lie on return from school, perhaps watching television or reading. This is ideally done on a hard surface, such as a blanket on the floor. The pre-school child can prone-lie after lunch but may need supervision to maintain the correct position.

The patient with flexion contractures of the hips requires extended periods of prone-lying to stretch the hip flexors. If possible, this should be carried out in school, one hour periods of prone-lying being alternated with one hour sitting throughout the day. If this is not practical, extra sessions of prone-lying should be fitted in before going to school and on return in the evening.

Posture and gait

Posture must be corrected at regular intervals so that bad habits are not formed. Similarly, gait requires correction as the tendency to limp, throw the leg or walk with flexed knees is all too frequently seen. Constant reminders to improve walking need to be given and the use of crutches may be necessary to aid this improvement. The child needs reminding to use his feet in the correct manner as he will often walk with a stiff gait, holding the foot rigid.

Splinting

Suitable splinting to rest the joints in a good position is essential. Splints may also be used to aid mobilisation of the patient and to correct deformity. The materials used for splinting are many (see Chapter 4).

REST SPLINTS

Neck involvement with loss of extension and limited lateral movements is helped by support from a collar, which prevents or assists correction of flexion and torticollis deformities. This can be made from foam, Plastazote or Orthoplast. Plastazote may require strengthening under the chin to maintain correction and Orthoplast, which is firmer, is preferable for torticollis correction.

The collar should be removed for eating to enable exercise of the temporomandibular joint and mandible.

Collapsed vertebrae may be seen in patients who have received high doses of corticosteroid drugs. These patients require a back brace as soon as they begin to mobilise. This can be a temporary one, made from Kramer wire and chiropody felt and bandaged into position, or a more permanent type of brace made from a plastic material. A Milwaukee brace may be necessary.

The wrists rapidly fall into flexion and sublux if left unsupported. A night rest splint holding the wrist in a maximum of 30° extension maintains a good position. This can be extended to support the fingers in slight flexion. The thumb should be supported on the palmar surface and held in opposition to the fingers. These splints can be made in plaster of Paris or plastic.

Knee involvement requires a back slab for night use, with the addition of a foot piece at right angles to the leg, if the ankle is also involved.

WORK SPLINTS AND SPLINTS TO AID MOBILITY

Splints to hold the wrist stable may be necessary to allow the child to carry out every day activities such as writing, drawing, etc. These can be made in plaster of Paris, but ideally should be made of plastic so that they can be washed as necessary. The thumb should be free to move in all directions and the splint should not extend too far into the palm to allow the metacarpophalangeal joints to flex fully.

When mobilising the child, it may be necessary to use a back slab or cylinder for one or both knees to gain stability of these joints. The back slab is used when there is weakness of the quadriceps muscles, but with slight flexion or lateral instability of the knee, it is preferable to use a cylinder. As muscle power increases the child is weaned off the splints.

Insoles can be inserted in the shoes to correct varus or valgus at the ankle and these can be extended to support the longitudinal arch. Acute pain in the ankle may respond to the application of double Tubigrip or strapping in a figure of eight pattern. If the pain fails to respond to this treatment, it may be necessary to seek the advice of an orthopaedic consultant, who may decide on a manipulation under anaesthesia followed by a period of time in a walking plaster. Extra care of the other joints must be taken if this is carried out, as strain is often thrown onto the hip and knee of the other side.

The metatarsal area is not often troublesome in the very young child but in the teenage patient can cause many problems. A metatarsal pad in the shoe or a metatarsal bar on the sole may relieve pain. Faradic foot baths and intrinsic exercises are given. Walking re-education may be required.

SERIAL SPLINTING

The dropped wrist is frequently seen in the patient who has not received any form of exercise or splinting. If the wrist is allowed to remain in fixed flexion, function of the fingers is impaired. A series of plaster of Paris splints can improve the position of the wrist.

The plaster of Paris is applied over stockinette and cotton wool padding. The forearm is held firmly by one hand, at the level of the ulnar styloid, and traction is applied to the wrist with the other hand. As the patient relaxes, the hand and wrist are pushed up into extension and the position is held by the plaster of Paris, which is applied round the wrist and between the thumb and index finger. Room is left in the palm for the fingers to flex at the metacarpophalangeal joints. This should be left on for 48 hours, then removed by splitting the plaster down the ulnar side of the splint, so that it can be slipped off over the thumb. The edges of the plaster can be tidied up and the splint reapplied with a bandage to hold it in position. Application of this splint, if carried out at the weekend, will not interfere with the exercise and hydrotherapy programme during the week and allows intensive physiotherapy to be continued to the wrists. A further splint can be applied at weekly intervals until a suitable correction has been achieved, when a more permanent plastic splint can be made to hold the wrist in the corrected position.

Flexion contractures of the knees often respond well to serial splinting. Traction is applied with one hand just above the malleoli and pressure on the medial side of the knee joint is applied with the other hand. The knee is held in plaster of Paris for 48 hours, then the splint is split down the lateral side and slipped off. After being tidied up the splint can be reapplied as a night splint. Further serial splints can be applied after a week's intensive physiotherapy until a satisfactory position is obtained. Care must be taken when pressure is applied to the area of the knee joint, as fractures in the supracondylar region have been known to occur. It must be remembered that the quadriceps muscles will be weak, so the patient may require a back slab or cylinder for walking until these are strengthened. Asymmetrical knee joint involvement may result in the unaffected leg being shorter than the affected leg necessitating a shoe raise on the unaffected side. This may only become obvious after serial splinting has straightened the affected knee.

Traction

Acute hip involvement requires prolonged bilateral skin traction in conjunction with twice daily hydrotherapy and three separate hourly periods of prone-lying. Sitting for meals may be allowed, but the remainder of the day and night should be spent flat, as the development of scoliosis is often seen in the child with hip disease. Mobilisation on a tricycle can begin when the hips have been pain free for at least two weeks. This enables the child to be mobile and relatively independent while increasing the movement in the hips and knees. Partial weight-bearing with crutches and night traction may need to be continued for many months to allow the hips to recover.

Chronic hip flexion contracture can be overcome with traction at night and extended periods of prone-lying, as described previously. Intensive hip and back extension exercises must be encouraged to gain the maximum benefit, and wheelchairs should only be used for transportation on long journeys. Tricycling is the method of transport which should be used by the child when not walking.

Hot, moist packs

The child with arthritis seems to prefer a moist heat and in addition to hydrotherapy and the use of a bath, the application of hot damp packs to any part of the body to relieve pain and muscle spasm can be used. These can be given prior to exercise to a specific joint or, as in the case of acute pain in the neck, may be used prior to gentle manual traction followed by active exercises if possible. They are also useful to relax the patient before the application of serial splints.

Wax

Patients find hot wax application beneficial prior to exercises for the individual joints of the fingers. The child is encouraged to make a full fist; a common error is to adduct the thumb across the palm in such a way that the index finger is unable to flex at the metacarpophalangeal joint. This must be corrected by holding the thumb away from the palm while a fist is formed and then allowing it to fold over the closed fingers.

Ice

Ice seems preferable to wax in the treatment of hot swollen hands. The patient with severe flexor tendon involvement of the fingers finds movement of the individual joints in the fingers easier after the application of a cold pack (Fig. 8.5).

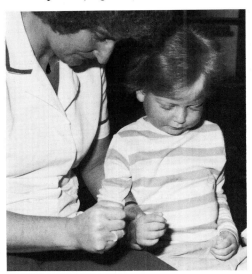

Fig. 8.5. Finger flexion exercises. Note the lack of flexion at the metacarpophalangeal joints.

Aids for daily living

These should be supplied as necessary to enable the patient to dress, undress, go to the toilet, etc. This aspect is particularly important for the teenage girls who need to be able to attend to their personal hygiene and cope with menstruation, in addition to looking after their appearance. Close co-operation with the occupational therapist is essential and functional assessments need to be carried out at regular intervals.

PARENTAL EDUCATION

Communication with the parents about the progress of their child and his treatment is necessary throughout his stay in hospital and as an out-patient. It is important that the parents understand the drug regime and the reasons for the administration of his medication. It is equally important that they understand the exercise and splinting programme and the reasons for it. The exercises are shown and demonstrated to the parents during the course of treatment in hospital so that they know what will be expected of them on the child's return home. The application of splints and traction must be explained. The child may need to attend the hospital for regular checks by the therapist to ensure that the exercises are being carried out correctly and daily, and that the splints are fitting properly and being worn. As the patient and parents become more able to carry out the management programme, the length of time between these attendances may be lengthened.

SCHOOLS

Some children may go to ordinary schools, others to schools for the physically handicapped. Some guidance for the teachers of those in ordinary schools is necessary; communication with the head teacher with a few guidelines such as whether the child can climb stairs, carry books etc., helps considerably in the reabsorption of the child into his normal school. Games are not usually allowed, but it may be possible for the child to join in with some of the non-impact games in the gymnasium. For those children attending a school for the physically handicapped a report to the physiotherapist is necessary to give up-to-date information about the child and his progress.

SURGERY

Prior to any surgery it is essential to gain the co-operation of the child and exercises must be started as soon as possible following surgery under the guidance of the orthopaedic consultant. The general scheme of exercises for all the joints should be continued and care about the position of the patient in bed at this time is of great importance. Splints should be worn to prevent flexion contractures and periods lying flat should be carried out during the day. Mobilisation should start as soon as possible.

SUMMARY

The treatment of children with arthritis is a long and difficult task, involving many years of routine exercises, splinting, medication and observation. There may be times when the disease appears inactive, but the joints and muscles can still become stiff and weak. It is essential that the patient continues his programme of exercises to remain as fit as possible at all times, so that in the event of a relapse of the disease he can perform the exercises and prevent muscle weakness and joint deformity. Encouragement from the medical and paramedical team and from his relatives and friends will help enormously in his attempts to achieve a normal life.

FURTHER READING

ALLIN R. E. & LAWTON S. (1977) The management of J.C.P. *Association of Paediatric Chartered Physiotherapists.*

ANSELL B. M. (1969) Still's disease. *Journal of the Royal College of Physicians,* **4,** 49–54.

ANSELL B. M. (1972) The management of juvenile chronic polyarthritis (Still's disease). *The Practitioner, Symposium on Rheumatological Remedies,* **208,** 91–100.

ANSELL B. M. (1973) Still's disease. *Nursing Times,* **59, 19** 596–600.

ANSELL B. M., WILLIAMS J. G. P., CHESHIRE L., LAWTON S. & HAINES R. E. J. (1972) Farnham Park modular splint system. *Rheumatology and Physical Medicine,* **11,** 334–335.

BYWATERS E. G. L. (1971) Still's disease in adults. *Annals of the Rheumatic Diseases,* **30,** 121–133.

HOUCHIN R. & CHESHIRE L. (1971) Splintage for ulnar deviation. *Occupational Therapy,* **34,** 9.

LAWTON D. S. (1974) Hand splinting in rheumatoid arthritis. *Occupational Therapy,* **37, 12** 219–226.

LAWTON D. S. & GOBB S. (1974) Children's functional assessment. *Occupational Therapy,* **37, 10** 175–177.

RENN G. (1976) Initial investigation into the effect of wrist splinting in children with Still's disease. *Occupational Therapy,* **39,** 9.

9 Ankylosing Spondylitis

Ankylosing spondylitis is one of the sero negative inflammatory arthropathy group of diseases; it is of unknown aetiology and unlike rheumatoid arthritis has a predilection for men rather than women in a ratio that is variously reported as between 7 and 5:1.

Typically it has an insidious onset, usually occurring in the second and third decades, although in a small proportion of cases symptoms may be present in the early teens. In a further small percent (less than 10%) the condition is associated with Still's disease. Ankylosing spondylitis results in bony ankylosis beginning with ossification of ligaments and tendons of the spine, particularly at junctions with bone. Ossification usually starts at the dorso-lumbar region. Around joints there is loss of cortex, and erosions with consequent widening of joint spaces. Later in the disease process there is sclerosis and finally ankylosis.

CLINICAL FEATURES

The patient usually presents with a history of low back pain, early morning stiffness, a general feeling of malaise and in some cases night back pain. There is no history of trauma and no radiation of pain into the legs, neither are there the sensory changes associated with prolapsed intervertebral disc lesions. More rarely, the patient first presents with pain and stiffness in a proximal joint but in this case a careful history will reveal a previous attack of low back pain that was insufficient to warrant medical advice.

On clinical examination, pain is elicited on compression of the sacro-iliac joints and lumbar spinal movement is restricted, particularly lateral flexion. There is also loss of the lumbar lordosis.

In later stages of the disease, the thoracic spine is involved and this is evidenced by loss of rotation and, with the costovertebral joints compromised, a restricted chest wall mobility. The cervical spine is also affected and the movements of lateral flexion and rotation are restricted early in the course of the disease. Peripheral joints, particularly the hip and shoulder, may be similarly affected by pain and loss of movement.

Where the disease runs its full course and treatment has not been effective, the patient may become very disabled and adopt a classical deformity (Fig. 9.1). The deformity is one of hip and knee flexion, loss of lumbar curve with gross kyphosis, loss of cervical curve and protrusion of the jaw. The natural history of the disease is one of slow progression of ankylosis, with long periods of remission interspersed by exacerbation and in many cases the disease is self-limiting.

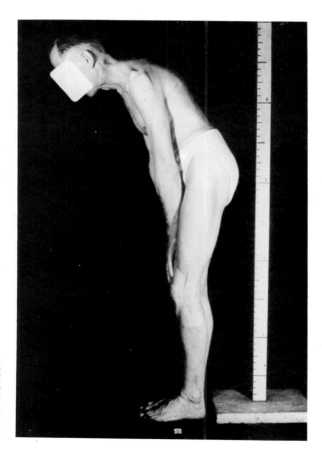

Fig. 9.1. Patient with advanced ankylosing spondylitis, attempting to stand erect. Note position of hands on thighs to maintain balance.

Table 9.1. Definition of ankylosing spondylitis according to the New York Criteria (Bennett and Wood, 1968).

Clinical criteria

1. Limitation of motion of the lumbar spine in all three planes – anterior flexion, lateral flexion and extension.

2. History of the presence of pain at the dorsolumbar junction or in the lumbar spine.

3. Limitation of chest expansion to 1 in (2.5 cm) or less measured at the level of fourth intercostal space.

Definite ankylosing spondylitis

1. Grade 3–4 bilateral sacro-iliitis with at least one clinical criterion; or

2. Grade 3–4 unilateral or Grade 2 bilateral sacro-iliitis with clinical criterion 1 or with both clinical criteria 2 and 3.

There are three cardinal signs of ankylosing spondylitis according to Bennett and Wood [1] (Table 9.1).

The X-ray changes of ankylosing spondylitis are characteristic and unmistakable in the advanced case; they are:

1. The formation of syndesmophytes, that is calcification of the annulus, distinguishable from osteophyte formation by the vertical formation of the calcification. It is this formation which together with the calcification of the longitudinal ligaments gives rise to the typical 'bamboo spine' appearance (Fig. 9.2).

2. Changes in the sacro-iliac joint – these show a progression from blurring of the joint with patchy osteoporosis and sclerosis to complete obliteration of the joint with ankylosis (Fig. 9.3).

3. The presence of new bone formation at the junction of the femoral head and neck in a 'ruff' formation.

Complications and associated disorders

The involvement of systems other than the musculoskeletal system is rare in ankylosing spondylitis but the following may occur.

Iritis

Cardiac – lone aortic incompetence

Ulcerative colitis

Associated psoriasis

Neurological involvement – may result from spinal fractures of which there is an increased incidence.

It is unusual for any of the above to prevent the patient from participating in active treatment, except of course where there is a fracture.

In a follow up study [2] of 222 cases it was reported that although there was functional impairment most patients continued to be fully

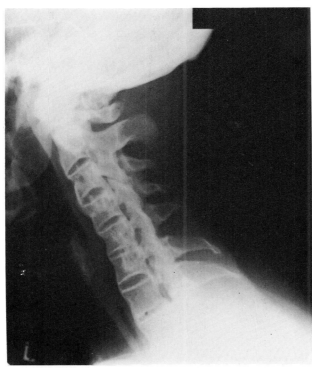

Fig. 9.2. Radiograph of cervical spine in patient with advanced ankylosing spondylitis.

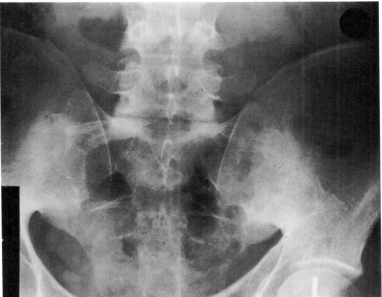

Fig. 9.3. Radiograph showing advanced sacro-iliitis in patient with ankylosing spondylitis.

employed and independent and the disease process did not appear to shorten life.

Blood tests

ESR – This may be raised during active phases of the disease but never reaches the high levels seen in rheumatoid arthritis.

HLA B27

This was initially thought to be a definitive test for ankylosing spondylitis. Brewerton [3], reported a 96% incidence in ankylosing spondylitis, with 4% in the control group, but a study by Grahame [4] showed that it was probably of more value clinically as an exclusion test.

TREATMENT

Drugs: Phenylbutazone
        Indomethacin

Surgery: Surgical intervention is rarely indicated in ankylosing spondylitis. However, where the disease is advanced and deformity is causing gross disablement total hip replacement may be undertaken. The physiotherapy required will be as described on p. 93, but these patients will require greater encouragement with breathing exercises and general mobilisation.

In rare circumstances spinal osteotomy may be necessary. Intensive chest physiotherapy is then needed to ensure adequate ventilation and respiratory toilet.

PHYSIOTHERAPY

The assessment of the patient with known ankylosing spondylitis may include some of the standard methods described earlier but in addition the following measurements should be made serially.

Posture
Spinal movement
Chest mobility and lung function

Posture

Since the postural deviations found in ankylosing spondylitis occur mainly in an antero-posterior direction, namely loss of lumbar curve and increased kyphosis with loss of cervical curve and protrusion, it is advisable to make objective measurements of these. In this unit a simple device, known as a spondylometer, is used. The spondylometer consists of an upright wooden post mounted at right angles to a wooden platform forming the base. The upright post is transected at two inch intervals by short rods which are movable in a horizontal direction. The upright and the rods are calibrated.

The patient stands on the base with his back to the upright, care being taken to ensure that at each measurement the medial malleoli of the tibia are at a fixed distance apart and the knees as straight as possible.

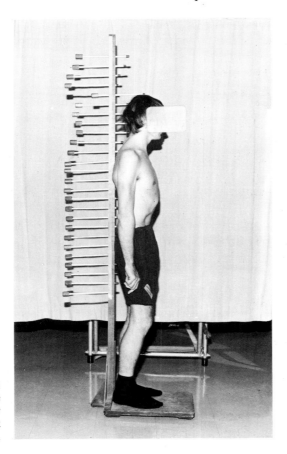

Fig. 9.4. Patient on spondylometer, note protrusion of the jaw and flexion deformity at knee.

The vertebral spinous processes are centred over the tips of the rods. The rods are then adjusted so that they just touch the spinous process. In the cervical region particular attention should be taken to ensure that the patient does not simply extend at the atlanto-axial joint with resultant protrusion; this is frequently the response to the verbal instruction to stand as straight as possible (Fig. 9.4).

Once the examiner is certain that the measurements are complete, the patient steps off the platform and a spinal profile is apparent. The information is recorded by plotting the figures on graph paper (Fig. 9.5).

These measurements should be recorded at six-monthly intervals.

PHOTOGRAPHY

It is very helpful to have photographic records of posture but this need only be repeated at two-yearly intervals to augment the objective

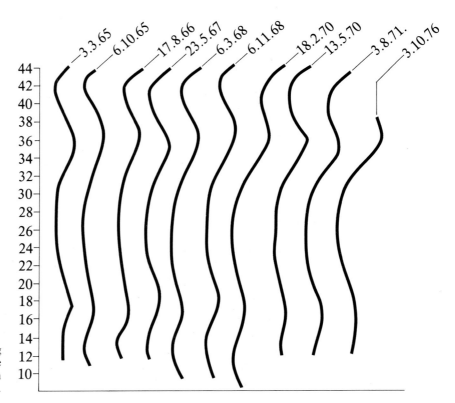

Fig. 9.5. Graph showing anteroposterior posture measured serially in patient (Mr M.).

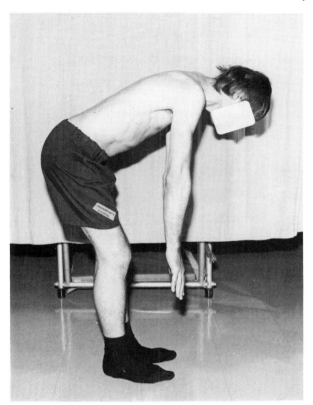

Fig. 9.6. Ankylosing spondylitic patient attempting forward flexion. Note inability to flex cervical spine, flat back and flexion deformity at knees.

measurements previously described. A simple lateral view is all that is necessary, although a further lateral view with the patient assuming the fully flexed, finger tip to toe position is helpful (Fig. 9.6).

Spinal movement

There are various methods for measuring spinal movement recorded in the literature and the method chosen depends on the degree of accuracy required, the degree of inter-observer error noted with each method and the availability of sophisticated equipment for measuring. Since the natural history of the ankylosing spondylitic patient requires that he is monitored over many years and will therefore be seen by many different observers, the following method is advocated and used in our clinic. It also has the advantage of not requiring expensive equipment.

The patient is asked to stand in the upright position with his back to the observer, with the medial malleoli a fixed distance apart, the arms in the anatomical position, the knees straight. The sacro-coccygeal position is located by palpation and the skin marked, similarly C7 is identified. A tape measure is used to measure the distance between these two points. The patient is then asked to flex his spine as far as possible and the distance is again measured. The measurement is then repeated with the spine in full extension. Lateral flexion is measured in a similar manner using the distance between the tip of the fingers and the floor.

Movement of the cervical spine is considered separately; forward flexion, extension, rotation and lateral flexion are recorded.

Combined hip and spinal movements are measured by asking the patient to flex his trunk as far as possible with the arms and hands reaching towards the floor, ensuring that the knees are maintained in the extended position. The distance recorded is that between tip of little finger and floor.

Other objective methods of measuring spinal mobility in ankylosing spondylitis are well documented in the literature [5, 6, 7, 8] but all require specific equipment.

Another method of measuring spinal mobility which has been found easy to use in an out-patient clinic and has good reproducibility with minimal inter- and intra-observer error is the Dunham Spondylometer [9]. This spondylometer was used in a study [10] to determine normagrams of spinal movement for normal subjects and a group of ankylosing spondylitic subjects measured over a period of 14 years.

PERIPHERAL JOINT MOVEMENT

This is measured using the standard techniques described on p. 22.

Any involvement of the temporomandibular joints should also be noted.

Lung function

The relatively early involvement of the costo-vertebral joints in the disease process makes careful spirometry and measurement of chest cage movement essential. It has been suggested that the spirogram may serve as an early diagnostic test for ankylosing spondylitis [11]. A 'reversed emphysema sign', that is impaired inspiratory flow rates, is demonstrated. Another study [12] reported similar findings but did not find any increased incidence of lung disease. A vitalograph machine is most useful but a more simple spirometer or peak flow device is adequate. Total vital capacity (FVC) is measured and a value obtained for the forced expiratory volume in one second (FEV_1). The resultant FEV_1/FVC ratio will be typical of restrictive lung disease.

Chest movement is measured at two levels, the ziphoid junction and nipple line on full inspiration and full expiration. The patient is measured in the standing position with the arms at the side. The measurement is recorded and the difference between the two measurements gives the value of excursion.

Studies [13] undertaken have shown the distribution of anterior, lateral spinal flexion and spinal extension in normal and ankylosing spondylitic patients and the correlations between these on chest expansion. The interpretation of these findings has importance in the design of exercise programmes.

Aims of physiotherapy

1. To maintain general mobility and posture
2. To maintain and improve physical endurance
3. To mobilise specific joints and prevent deformity
4. To relieve pain
5. To advise or counsel

Methods

EXERCISE

Although these patients may require individual instruction in exercise, they are best treated in groups (Fig. 9.7). The exercises should be simple, limited in number and such that the patient is encouraged to perform them daily himself. This cannot be emphasised enough, for as with the bronchiectatic patient, the degree to which management is successful will depend on the patient's acceptance of a daily treatment routine. In ankylosing spondylitis, unlike many of the other rheumatological diseases, an aggressive approach to physical exercise is essential. The exercise programme is designed to improve or maintain posture, physical endurance and mobility rather than strength, since muscle weakness is not a significant feature of the disease.

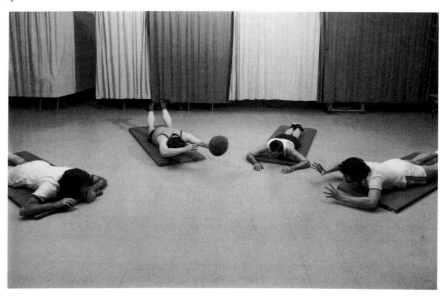

Fig. 9.7. Class activities for ankylosing spondylitis.

The advantages of a class are:

1. The support given by members to each other
2. Shared problems – providing a good medium for patients' education about the disease process
3. Competitive and motivational aspects
4. Improvement in physical endurance

A typical class is outlined below:

Supine lying

Relaxation—leading into posture correction and an awareness of position
Static quadriceps contractions
Static gluteal contraction
Straight leg raising

Crook lying

Pelvic tilting
Diaphragmatic breathing exercises
Arm elevation maintaining the thoracic spine in contact with the floor and with attention to the position of the cervical spine
Neck rotation

Prone lying

Alternate hip and leg extension
Bilateral leg extension
Arms at the side – shoulder retraction, head and shoulders extension
Bilateral leg abduction
Trunk side flexion
Arms extended, head, neck and trunk extension, a medicine ball may be lifted to offer resistance.

Sitting

Breathing exercises
Posture correction
Neck rotation and side flexion
Trunk rotation

Standing

Posture correction
Alternate knee and hip flexion to 90° at increasing frequency
Breathing exercises

Activities

Basket ball
Volley ball
Throughout the class activities it may be necessary for either the activity or the starting position to be modified by the use of pillows to make it possible for all members of the group to participate. It is important that each member does participate in the whole class.

Spring circuit

A spring circuit is used in the 'warm up' period before the class. The emphasis is on trunk extension (Fig. 9.8). In the department at Hammersmith Hospital a weekly class for ankylosing spondylitic patients has been held in the evening for the past 25 years and long term follow up of patients has therefore been possible. It is our impression that the class is important in the overall physical management.

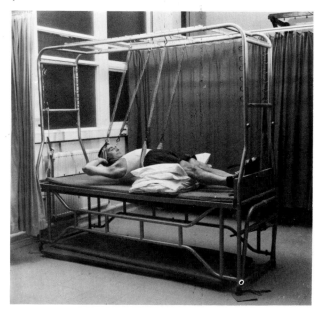

Fig. 9.8. Spring resistance exercise for hip and trunk extension.

HEAT AND MOBILISATION FOR SPECIFIC JOINT PROBLEMS

When specific joints are in a state of exacerbation, either vertebral or peripheral, Maitland mobilisation techniques are used with good effect.

It is sometimes necessary to give short intensive courses of exercise therapy when the patient presents in acute exacerbation. In these circumstances techniques of proprioceptive neuromuscular facilitation are most useful, in particular hold relax, rhythmic stabilisation and slow reversals.

The use of forms of heat may be contraindicated, if the patient has received empirical radiotherapy (a treatment less frequently used now), and in any case is of doubtful benefit. Damp hot packs may be helpful in relieving pain from muscle spasm.

Short term beneficial effects of physiotherapy on cervical movement in ankylosing spondylitis have been demonstrated [14].

HYDROTHERAPY

This is of benefit in the general management of the ankylosing spondylitic both for individual treatment and group therapy [15].

THE USE OF SPLINTS

Splints, either corrective or night rest, are contraindicated. Prevention of deformity is best achieved by exercise.

Advice or counselling

The insidious manner in which ankylosis progresses over many years makes it imperative that the patient understands the nature of the disease and is encouraged to take an aggressive attitude to exercise. Patients are encouraged to take up sports such as squash and swimming. An understanding of the importance of posture is essential. The physiotherapist should ensure that she discusses the patient's occupational, sitting and sleeping posture, and where necessary suggests alternatives or modifications.

The National Organisation for Ankylosing Spondylitis publishes helpful advice and where indicated patients may be encouraged to join this group.

Case history

Mr M. 40 years old (Table 9.2 and see Fig. 9.5).

January 1965

First presented at this hospital with low back pain, with a previous history of episodes of back pain with some radiation into left leg, for which he had received traditional physiotherapy and a corset at another hospital.

March 1965

Ankylosing spondylitis diagnosed. Physiotherapy assessment and attendance at ankylosing spondylitis class. Patient attended regularly until June 1968. During this period the disease remained active and the patient suffered intermittent bouts of neck pain, pain in the left hip and knee and iritis. Drug therapy consisted of indomethacin and phenyl butazolodine.

March 1969

Patient no longer attending class because of changed social circumstances and became increasingly less vigilant about home exercise programme.

February–May 1970

Attended ankylosing spondylitis class again.

Table 9.2.
Name: Mr M.

No.

Hammersmith Hospital
Postgraduate Medical School of London
Physiotherapy Department

Ankylosing Spondylitis
Progress Report

Dates	3.3.65	6.10.65	17.8.66	23.5.67	20.3.68	6.11.68	18.2.70	13.5.70	3.8.71	76
Spine:										
Vertebra prominens to sacro-coccygeal junction										
a) straight	22½ (inches)	22½	22½	22½	22½	22½	22½	23½	23½	23½
b) flexed	26	26	26½	27	26½	26½	24	25¼	24¼	24¼
c) extended	21½	20	21½	22¼	22	22	22	22¾	22½	23¼
Combined spine and hip flexion:										
Standing forward bending from tip of little finger to floor	8¾	able to touch floor	able to touch floor	4	3	7	23	9½	12	10
Stride lying distance between malleoli	42½	44	42½	42	44	40	38½	36½	41	34½
Chest at level of xyphoid process										
a) inspiration	34¼	34¼	36½	37	35¼	36	35	37	37¼	37¼
b) expiration	32¼	32¼	34	35¼	33¼	34½	34	36	36¼	36¼
c) expansion	1¾	2¼	2½	1¾	2	1½	1	1	1	1
Shoulders										
Hips										
Vital capacity	3200	3300	2950	3200	3300	2000	2000	2100	2700	2350
Physiotherapist										

Table 9.3.
Name: Mr T.   No.

Hammersmith Hospital
Postgraduate Medical School of London
Physiotherapy Department

Ankylosing Spondylitis
Progress Report

Dates	5.12.75	13.12.76	15.2.78	28.2.79
Spine:				
Vertebra prominens to sacro-coccygeal junction				
a) straight	59cms	57	54	54
b) flexed	68	64	67.5	66
c) extended	58	54	52	49½
Combined spine and hip flexion:				
Standing forward bending from tip of little finger to floor	18	8	4	Touches floor easily
Stride lying distance between malleoli	84	98	100	99
Chest at levels of xyphoid process				
a) inspiration	84	86	90.5	88
b) expiration	79½	78	82.5	79½
c) expansion	4½	8	8	8.5
Shoulders				
Hips				
Vital capacity				
Physiotherapist				

February 1971
Received empirical radiotherapy because of unremitting pain.
February 1971–1979
Patient made only very infrequent attendances at the class but did attend for assessment on two occasions. Patient now has difficulty in walking with pain in both hips, left more than right, with radiation to the knees.

Case history

Mr B.
1958
Referred to Hammersmith Hospital with a diagnosis of ankylosing spondylitis, aged 22 years. Empirical radiotherapy given to cervical spine, thoracic spine and lumbar spine. Patient assessed and started attending ankylosing spondylitis class. Attended regularly until 1962.
1962
Patient stopped attending class because of change in place of employment, but re-assessed at regular intervals.
1967
Exacerbation neck pain and pain in right hip.
1976
Recommended regular attendance at class.

Case history

Mr T. 31 year old male (Table 9.3).
December 1975
Admitted to hospital with dyspnoea at rest and arthritis involving the small joints of the hand, wrist, shoulder, lumbar spine and ankles. Diagnosed as ankylosing spondylitis and acute pericarditis.
Treatment
    Drugs: Indomethacin
                      Steroids
    Physiotherapy: General mobilising exercises and participation in class.
February 1976
Steroids stopped.
    Out-patient attendance of ankylosing spondylitis class continued to date. Patient plays tennis, squash and cricket regularly. The improvement in range of motion and posture are demonstrated by the serial measurements shown.

REFERENCES

[1] BENNETT P. H. & WOOD P. H. N. (1968) Diagnostic criteria for ankylosing spondylitis. *Population Studies of the Rheumatic Diseases*, p. 456. International Congress Series, No. 148.

[2] WILKINSON M. & BYWATERS E. G. L. (1958) Clinical features and course of ankylosing spondylitis. *Annals of the Rheumatic Diseases*, **17**, 209–227.

[3] BREWERTON D. A., CAFFREY M., HART F. D., JAMES D. C. O., NICHOLLS A. & STURROCK R. D. (1973) Ankylosing spondylitis and HL-A27. *Lancet*, **i**, 904–907.

[4] GRAHAME R., KENNEDY L. & WOOD P. H. N. (1975) HL-A27 and the diagnosis of back problems. *Rheumatology and Rehabilitation*, **14**, 168–172.

[5] LOEBL W. Y. (1967) Measurement of spinal posture and range of spinal movement. *Annals of Physical Medicine*, **9**, 103.

[6] MACRAE I. F. & WRIGHT V. (1969) Measurement of back movement. *Annals of the Rheumatic Diseases*, **28**, 584–589.

[7] MOLL J. M. H., LIYANAGE S. P. & WRIGHT V. (1972) An objective clinical method to measure lateral spinal flexion. *Rheumatology and Physical Medicine*, **11**, 225.

[8] MOLL J. M. H. & WRIGHT V. (1971) Normal range of spinal mobility. An objective clinical study. *Annals of the Rheumatic Diseases*, **30**, 381–386.

[9] DUNHAM W. F. (1949) Ankylosing spondylitis – measurement of hip and spine movements. *British Journal of Physical Medicine*, **12**, 126.

[10] STURROCK R. D., WOJTULEWSKI J. A. & HART F. D. (1973) Spondylometry in a normal population and in ankylosing spondylitis. *Rheumatology and Rehabilitation*, **12**, 135–142.

[11] BASS B. H. & WENLEY W. G. (1961) The spirogram in ankylosing spondylitis – the 'reversed emphysema' sign. *Annals of Physical Medicine*, **6,3**, 105–108.

[12] HART F. D., EMERSON P. A. & GREGG I. (1963) Thorax in ankylosing spondylitis. *Annals of the Rheumatic Diseases*, **22**, 11–17.

[13] MOLL J. M. H. & WRIGHT V. (1973) The pattern of chest and spinal mobility in ankylosing spondylitis. *Rheumatology and Rehabilitation*, **12**, 115–134.

[14] O'DRISCOLL S. L., JAYSON M. I. V. & BADDELEY H. (1978) Neck movements in ankylosing spondylitis and their responses to physiotherapy. *Annals of the Rheumatic Diseases*, **37**, 64–66.

[15] HARRISON R. A. & DIXON A. S. J. (1975) Group treatment for ankylosing spondylitis. *Rehabilitation*, British Health Care and Technology. Health and Social Services Journal.

10 Systemic Lupus Erythematosus

Mrs O. M. Scott

INTRODUCTION

Systemic lupus erythematosus (SLE) was one of the least well known of the connective tissue diseases but it has recently been the subject of extensive research and clinical studies. It is a widespread systemic disease which most commonly affects young women in their late teens and early twenties and takes a typically cyclic course of acute exacerbation followed by variable periods of remission. It used to have a grave prognosis of rapid progression to renal failure and death.

It is generally accepted that the manifestations of the disease with its extensive involvement of many organs are directly related to the disturbance of the immune mechanisms of the body, and the resulting formation of immune complexes.

The discovery by Hargraves and his co-workers of the lupus erythematosus (LE) cell in bone marrow in 1948 [1], and the introduction of adrenocortical therapy shortly afterwards led to a considerable change in the pessimistic outlook. The development of sophisticated tests for measuring the levels of anti DNA antibody and serum complement (see p. 186) in the blood have improved the diagnostic procedures and provided laboratory tests which are used to monitor the activity of the disease and its response to clinical management. The disease can be diagnosed earlier and milder forms are being recognised.

INCIDENCE

Studies of the incidence of SLE show that the male/female ratio is 1:9

and that the disease appears to be more prevalent in Negro than Caucasian populations.

Fessel, in a study in San Francisco [2], found that one case of SLE occurred in approximately 2000 people, but that the prevalence for black women between the ages of 15–64 was one case in 245. He showed that the disease is often benign and that 90% of the diagnosed cases had survived for over 10 years. SLE is no longer the rare and fatal disease that it was once considered.

AETIOLOGY

Sudden onset of the acute symptoms of SLE can be associated with recent exposure to sunlight/UVR and may result in a violent skin reaction and other symptoms of the disease. A similar reaction has been observed on taking certain drugs, and there appears to be a particular association with tetanus antitoxin, antibiotics and gold injections, or the patient may relate the symptoms to a recent sore throat or cold.

The aetiology of SLE has not yet been established and three principal causes are currently suggested:

1. Immunological
2. Infective/viral
3. Genetic

The proposition is that SLE is an immunological or more probably an autoimmunological disease. This means, by definition, a disease which results from the reaction between an auto-antigen and an auto-antibody resulting in tissue damage and clinical manifestations.

The evidence which supports this theory is that patients with lupus have an exceptional ability to form antinuclear antibodies and it is suggested that these antibodies of which the LE cell is an IgG antibody are the result of an auto-immune mechanism. Other workers suggest that there are certain inherited predisposing factors towards developing the disease, while others support the evidence of viral infection causing the raised levels of antibodies.

DIAGNOSIS

Although SLE may present with one or two features only, for purposes of classification, the American Rheumatism Association have published a list of criteria, of which at least four should be present [3]. These criteria have been criticised as being too rigid and are in the process of being revised.

American Rheumatism Association Preliminary Criteria for classification of SLE:

1. Facial lupus (butterfly rash)
2. Discoid lupus
3. Raynaud's phenomenon
4. Alopecia
5. Photosensitivity
6. Oral/nasal ulceration
7. Arthritis without deformity
8. LE cells × 2
9. Chronic false-positive tests for syphilis
10. Profuse proteinuria greater than 3.5 gm/day
11. Cellular casts
12. Pleurisy/pericarditis
13. Psychosis/convulsions
14. Haemolytic anaemia/leucopenia/thrombocytopaenia

A number of clinical studies have now been published based on these criteria and they provide comparative studies of the clinical features of the disease (Table 10.1).

Table 10.1. Cumulative major clinical manifestations of SLE in 4 studies [4]

	Grigor *et al.* (1978) 50 patients %	Lee *et al.* (1977) 100 patients %	Estes and Christian (1971) 150 patients %	Dubois *et al.* (1974) 520 patients %
Skin lesions	84	86.3	81	71.5
Raynaud's phenomenon	32	45.4	21	18.4
Alopecia	64	38.2	37	21.0
Oral ulcers	34	29.0	7	9.1
Arthritis	98	61.8	95	91.9
Nephritis	40	49.0	53	46.1
Pleurisy	52	30.9	48	45.0
Pericarditis	20	24.5	38	30.5
Neuropsychiatric	50	40.0	59	25.5

Clinical picture

The clinical picture of SLE can be very variable at onset, and this variability of presentation continues throughout the course of the disease. Skin and musculoskeletal involvement are the most frequently recorded manifestations. The incidence of neuropsychiatric involvement should be noted, and it is suggested that as many as two-thirds of all cases may have neuropsychiatric involvement.

The patient seen during an active phase of the disease is generally unwell and there may be a high fever of a cyclic type, a marked facial rash, and considerable muscle pain and weakness. Associated with this there may be great difficulty in performing simple physical tasks and an overall mental depression. In general, patients are managed on an outpatient basis, only being admitted for initial diagnosis or at a later stage if the disease becomes so active that the patient cannot be managed satisfactorily at home.

Skin and mucous membrane

One of the best known symptoms of SLE is the butterfly rash which extends from both cheeks across the bridge of the nose. It can occur after exposure to the sun but it is often transitory.

Many other skin conditions are associated with the disease and small areas of vasculitis are seen, often in the palms and around the nail beds.

Alopecia or hair loss may be severe and distressing, although some patients notice only slight patchy hair loss and an associated new growth of short hairs. Examination of the dermal-epidermal functions reveals increased deposition of gamma globulins and patients with SLE frequently comment on the patchy discolouration of their skin; this is a distinct sign of vasculitis [5].

Bone and joint involvement

Estes and Christian [6] found that almost every patient at some time complained of joint pain during the course of the disease. The joint involvement is commonly symmetrical and associated with marked synovitis and it occurs especially in the small joints. The pain and discomfort is usually eased with salicylates and X-rays very rarely show erosions.

A small number of patients develop joint deformity, probably because of joint capsule laxity. The hands can show the typical deformities of rheumatoid arthritis with MCP and wrist joint involvement, joint subluxation, ulnar deviation and 'swan neck' – so-called Jaccoud's arthritis – but even in these cases X-rays do not show erosive changes (Fig. 10.1).

Avascular (aseptic) necrosis was reported in 8% of the 110 cases reviewed by Lee *et al.* [7] and this figure agrees with other series. It appears

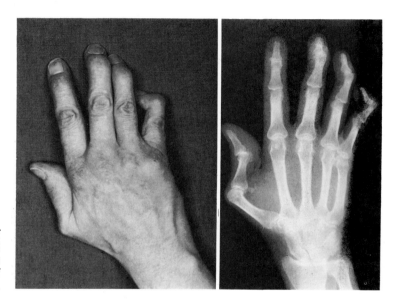

Fig. 10.1. Right hand of patient with SLE showing characteristic changes. Note absence of erosions on radiograph.

most commonly to affect the femoral heads but can occur elsewhere, for example in the humeral heads and the small bones of the hands and feet. It is often associated with high levels of steroid therapy. Patients may complain of severe localised pain months before X-ray changes can be identified. Treatment is initially conservative, and includes judicious use of rest splints, bed rest and later, where appropriate, walking aids should be provided. The symptoms may regress or the condition may be insidiously progressive and result in joint destruction, loss of mobility and eventually orthopaedic intervention and the insertion of prosthetic replacements may become necessary. This feature is almost certainly due to steroid therapy and not the underlying disease, and may become less frequent as more conservative therapy is accepted (Fig. 10.2).

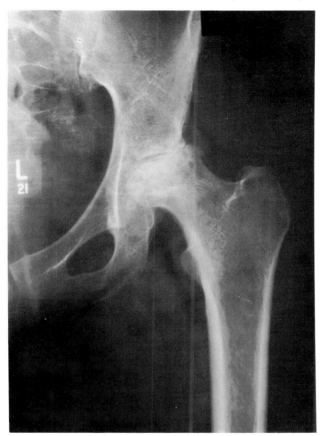

Fig. 10.2. Radiograph of hip in patient with SLE showing collapse of femoral head.

Arteries

Localisation of immune complexes not destroyed by the reticulo-endothelial system results in inflammation of small and medium sized arteries [5]. Vasculitis is a conspicuous feature of SLE accounting for many of the skin conditions associated with the disease, the multiple organ involvement and the pathology of the serosal membranes.

Muscles

Myalgia, arthralgia and arthritis are often grouped together under various headings in reported clinical studies. Patients, however, readily distinguish between localised joint pain and generalised tenderness of muscles associated with muscle pathology. Dubois [8] reported that

48.2% of the 520 cases he reviewed complained of myalgia and tenderness and that this was most marked in the deltoid and quadriceps muscles, and was associated with generalised muscle weakness. A recent study of 10 patients admitted to this unit for diagnosis and management of SLE showed a significant reduction in voluntary muscle force ($p < 0.001$) and an alteration of response to varying rates of electrical stimulation when compared with a control group [9].

Early muscle symptoms may be transitory and similar to the early morning stiffness well known in rheumatoid arthritis, and may account for the apparent lassitude and reluctance to move often observed in the recently diagnosed cases of SLE.

Alteration in muscle structure is not uncommon in SLE and histological examination [10] has revealed a number of different lesions. Estes and Christian [6] report myositis involving the proximal musculature, confirmed by muscle biopsy, electromyographic studies and elevation of serum creatine phosphokinase in seven of their 150 patients. It is necessary to distinguish between the pathological changes associated with a steroid-induced myopathy and those of a true inflammatory myositis which will respond to raised levels of steroid administration. Cases of steroid myopathy in SLE are possibly less frequent than is suggested in the literature.

PHYSIOTHERAPY

Inflammatory myositis is characterised by a generalised muscle tenderness which is usually relieved with raised levels of steroids, but some patients have developed marked pain with loss of extensibility in selected muscle groups, e.g. wrist and finger flexors, and present with an inability to fully extend the wrist and fingers resulting in a very disabling loss of hand function. Careful splinting provides maintenance of a functional position and relief of pain until the acute symptoms subside (Fig. 10.3a, b).

The aim of physiotherapy is to maintain and, if possible, increase muscle strength. Active resisted exercises are used to facilitate muscle activity. It is important to monitor the effects of alterations in drug and physical therapy. Following the initial increase of steroids, which can be as high as 60–80 mg/day, the steroids are gradually reduced and it is usually found that with active rehabilitation the muscle strength can be enhanced.

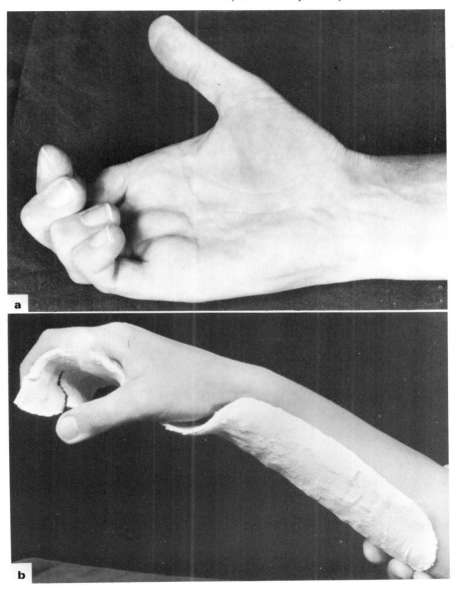

Fig. 10.3. (a) Patient attempting finger extension, which is prevented by flexor tightness. (b) Stretch plaster used for correction.

Renal involvement

Estimations of the incidence of renal pathology in patients with SLE is now as high as 80% [7], though the true incidence of significant disease is probably far lower. Investigations by light microscopy of biopsy specimens suggest that there are three main forms of kidney involvement: focal proliferative, diffuse proliferative, and membranous nephritis, although in the early stages reversion and transition between the types of lesion have been reported. A new pathologic form, mesangial lupus nephritis, has been identified which is often reversible and can be present without any clinical sign.

The deposition of immune complexes is now widely accepted as the cause of renal changes in SLE. The various histological changes may result either from differing immune responses to varying quantities of immune complexes, or from patients having different host responses to similar complexes. The survival rate of patients with lupus nephritis has markedly improved but renal disease is still a major cause of morbidity and mortality and in order to determine the probable prognosis it is necessary to determine the nature of the histology. Patients with membranous lupus nephritis have a relatively good prognosis and remission can occur, but for patients with diffuse proliferative nephritis the prognosis is grave and severe hypertension is followed by renal failure and death within months. Focal proliferative nephritis has a substantially benign course but transition to diffuse proliferative nephritis or to membranous forms is reported and it is suggested that focal and diffuse proliferative nephritis may be different phases of the same process [11].

Nervous system

The extent of neurological abnormalities in SLE is considerable and ranges from central disorders of mental function and seizures, to cranial nerve involvement, paresis and peripheral neuropathy.

Depression and psychosis occur frequently [6] and may be a very early symptom of the disease requiring considerable care and sensitivity in management, It is still sometimes in error thought to be a reaction to the diagnosis or to corticosteroid therapy. The psychoses include organic mental syndromes, manifesting as disorientation, and hallucinations, disorders of perception, memory or intellectual function and some patients complain of severe headaches of a migranous type.

Lee *et al.* [7] found that major neuropsychiatric manifestations occurred in 40% of patients and Baker [12], in a survey of 17 patients, found that 42% had serious psychiatric problems as a complication of SLE. The latter stated in his conclusion that psychiatric episodes do not represent an intensification of psychopathology present before the onset of the disease, and that SLE is not merely acting as a non-specific stress to predisposed individuals.

Epilepsy has been reported [13] in 17–50% of patients with CNS lupus and most commonly occurs during exacerbation of the disease. Isolated cranial nerve involvement occurs in 5–33% and may be sudden in onset, intermittent diplopia is common and recurrent transient ptosis. Hemiplegia and paraplegia occur occasionally. Peripheral neuritis, although less common than in rheumatoid arthritis, was observed in 7% of the 150 patients studied by Estes and Christian [6]; it is usually both symmetrical and sensory. Disorders of voluntary movement have been reported, chorea is most common but cerebellar ataxia has been observed.

It is suggested [5] that immune complex deposition in the cerebral vasculature accounts for some of the neuropathology. In this unit, EEG studies show the most frequent abnormal findings and of 39 patients admitted for 48 hours of planned investigations, abnormal EEG's were recorded in 10 of the 11 patients who had neuropsychiatric manifestations.

Pulmonary involvement

In recent investigation in this hospital, 30 patients were assessed for respiratory symptoms, and evidence was found of pulmonary involvement in 89% [14]. Defects in gas transfer, the carbon monoxide diffusing capacity, was found in 24 patients and in 13 patients the total lung capacity was below 80% of the predicted value.

Pleurisy is one of the most commonly recorded manifestations and was present in 50% of the patients reviewed by Estes and Christian [6], and in 40% it was accompanied by a small pleural effusion. It is frequently the cause of persistent localised chest pain and results in dyspnoea and shallow breathing.

Lupus pneumonia may cause recurrent atelectasis. There are diffuse pulmonary infiltrates and a non-bacterial sputum which does not respond to antibiotics, but does respond to steroids. One of the more frequent radiographic findings in such patients is a gradual elevation of the diaphragm and loss of the costophrenic angle leading to 'small lungs'. This progressive lung 'shrinkage' [14] may be caused by weakness of the respiratory muscles, in particular of the diaphragm, and may be part of a generalised myopathy (Fig. 10.4).

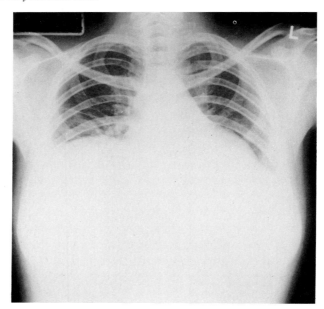

Fig. 10.4. Radiograph anteroposterior view of chest in patient with SLE, showing high diaphragm and 'small lungs'.

A 20-year-old secretary (Miss W.) with clinically very active SLE was admitted to hospital in December 1975. She was very unwell with a cyclic temperature up to 104°F and had marked musculoskeletal involvement and vasculitis and complained of shortness of breath. On the 8th January 1976 she developed marked pleuritic pain radiating from her left side. For the next five months she had continual acute exacerbation with increasing diminution of lung volumes, raised diaphragm, generalised muscle pain and weakness, despite treatment with high levels of systemic steroids (up to 80 mg/day). Serial recordings were made of lung function and muscle strength. Physical management included breathing exercises, IPPB to try to facilitate normal basal chest movement, and active mobilisation during periods of remission. On discharge, 1st July 1976, she was still very unwell and was readmitted on the 23rd August 1976. She managed to return to work on the 1st January 1977 and was reassessed on the 8th August 1977. Following this she gradually improved, and at her latest assessment was well, at work and on no therapy (Fig. 10.5).

Where there is pulmonary involvement the aim of treatment is to obtain the best possible lung function. Breathing exercises are given to

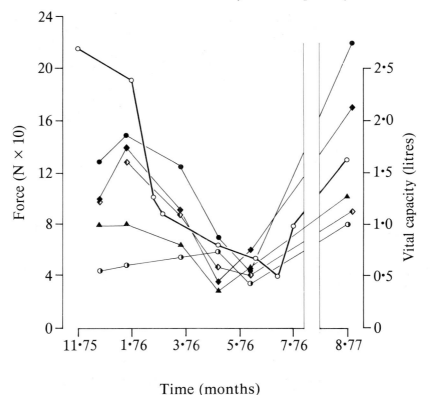

Fig. 10.5. The relationship of serial measurements of selected muscle groups and vital capacity of a patient (Miss W.) with SLE admitted to hospital December 1975–July 1976 and on re-assessment 18 months later.

o Vital capacity ◇ Hip flexors (R)
● Foot dorsiflexors (R) ▲ Shoulder abductors (R)
◆ Quadriceps (L) ◓ Wrist extensors (R)

encourage diaphragmatic breathing and lateral costal expansion of the thorax. In a very severe case, IPPB may be used to re-educate the breathing pattern or to aid mobilisation of secretions if they are present.

Cardiac involvement

Pericarditis is a common cardiac lesion, occurring in 20–30% of patients with systemic lupus. Patients complain of a persistent substernal pain and there is a slight enlargement of the heart shadow on X-ray. Myocarditis also occurs and is associated with tachycardia and abnormal ECG recordings.

Drug therapy

The introduction of corticosteroids in the 1950's substantially altered the prognosis for patients with systemic lupus. The current trend is to control the activity of the disease on the lowest possible level of steroids (average daily dose 7.5 mg/day). Prolonged high dosages of greater than 20 mg/day are only necessary in a very few patients and this may account for the fewer side-effects observed of bone necrosis, steroid myopathy and serious infections.

Aspirin, indomethacin and proprionic acid derivatives are used to control fever, joint and muscle pain, and serositis, and immuno-suppressive drugs are used particularly in the management of lupus nephritis.

Serial measurements used in monitoring of SLE

Two serological tests, DNA binding and serum complement estimations, are used to monitor the level of activity of the disease.

In most patients raised DNA binding levels in raised DNA antibody levels indicate increased generalised activity [15], where serum complement levels are used to monitor renal involvement and lowered values indicate active renal disease.

Physical parameters found to be of value include:

1. Measurement of force output of muscle groups using a myometer
2. Estimations of functional ability – grip strength/walking time
3. Simple lung function tests – forced expiratory volume (FEV_1) and vital capacity (VC)
4. Muscle function tests (see p. 7)

PROGNOSIS

This has considerably improved and the causes of death have altered. The outlook for patients with CNS involvement and renal disease is still grave, but death occurs more frequently from infection, vascular complications and malignant neoplasms [16].

REFERENCES

[1] HARGRAVES M. M., RICHMOND H. & MORTON R. (1948) Presentation of two bone marrow elements: the tart cell and the 'L.E.' cell. *Proceedings of Mayo Clinic*, **23**, 25.

[2] FESSEL W. J. (1974) Systemic lupus erythematosus in the community. *Archives of Internal Medicine*, **134**, 1027–1035.

[3] THE ARTHRITIS FOUNDATION (1971) Preliminary criteria for the classification of systemic lupus erythematosus. *Bulletin on the Rheumatic Diseases*, **9**, 643–648.

[4] GRIGOR R., EDMONDS J., LEWKONIA R., BRESNIHAN B. & HUGHES G. R. V. (1978) Systemic lupus erythematosus. A prospective analysis. *Annals of the Rheumatic Diseases*, **37**, 121–128.

[5] HUGHES G. R. V. (1977) *Connective Tissue Diseases*. Blackwell, Oxford.

[6] ESTES D. & CHRISTIAN C. L. (1971) The natural history of systemic lupus erythematosus by prospective analysis. *Medicine*, **50**, 85–95.

[7] LEE P., UROWITZ M. B., BOOKMAN A. M., KOEHLER B. E., SMYTHE H. A., GORDON D. A. & OGRYZLO M. A. (1977) Systemic lupus erythematosus. *Quarterly Journal of Medicine*, **46**, 181, 1–32.

[8] DUBOIS E. L. (1974) *Lupus Erythematosus*. 2nd Ed., Ch. 9, p. 262. University of California Press, Los Angeles.

[9] GRAHAM O. & HYDE S. A. (1978) The clinical application of quantitative muscle testing. *Proceedings of the 8th International Congress of Physical Therapy*.

[10] ADAMS R. D. (1975) *Diseases of Muscle*. 3rd Ed., Ch. 7, p. 363. Harper and Row, Maryland.

[11] APPEL G. B., SILVA F. G., PIRANI C. L., MELTZER J. I. & ESTES D. (1978) Renal involvement in SLE. *Medicine*, **57**, 371–409.

[12] BAKER M. (1973) Psychopathology in SLE. Psychiatric observations. *Seminars in Arthritis and Rheumatism*, **3**, 95–125.

[13] BENNETT R., HUGHES G. R. V., BYWATERS E. G. L. & HOLT P. J. L. (1972) Neuropsychiatric problems in SLE. *British Medical Journal*, **iv**, 342–345.

[14] GIBSON G. J., EDMONDS J. P. & HUGHES G. R. V. (1977) Diaphragm function and lung involvement in systemic lupus erythematosus. *American Journal of Medicine*, **63**, 926–932.

[15] LIGHTFOOT R. W. & HUGHES G. R. V. (1976) Significance of persisting serological abnormalities in systemic lupus erythematosus. *Arthritis and Rheumatism*, **19**, 837–843.

[16] DUBOIS E. L., WIERZCHOWIECKI M., COX M. B. & WEINER J. M. (1974) Duration and death in systemic lupus erythematosus. *Journal of the American Medical Association*, **227**, 1399–1402.

11 Polymyositis and Dermatomyositis

There are a group of conditions known collectively as inflammatory myopathies; polymyositis and dermatomyositis form part of this group. In some conditions the myositis is of known cause, e.g. bacterial or viral origin, but in pure polymyositis and dermatomyositis the aetiology is unknown, although they are increasingly associated with the connective tissue disorders.

The overlap between polymyositis and dermatomyositis is such that it was not until the late nineteenth century that two separate entities were delineated and only in 1954 that Walton and Adams [1] produced a classification that is now widely accepted. Many other classifications have been produced [2, 3] but for clarity in this chapter the following is used:

Classification

1. Pure polymyositis
2. Polymyositis with some evidence of other connective tissue disorders or a slight rash
3. Severe connective tissue disease with incidental myositis
4. Dermatomyositis
    a. Adult
        i. without malignancy
        ii. with malignancy
    b. Childhood

Although this classification is used, it must be emphasised that it is arbitrary since the clinical presentation and the tempo of the disease process are so variable, ranging from acute to chronic, that during the course of an illness a patient may change from one diagnostic category to another (Table (11.1).

Table 11.1. Percentage of clinical signs and symptoms in 133 cases of polymyositis. (From Barwick and Walton [4].)

	%
Musculature	
1. Weakness	
Proximal (arms)	99
(legs)	80
Distal	35
Neck flexors	65
Dysphagia	62
Facial muscles	5
Extraocular muscles	2
2. Pain or tenderness	48
3. Contractures	35
4. Atrophy	35
Skin	
1. Typical 'heliotrope' rash	40
2. Atypical rash	20
Other	
1. Raynaud's phenomenon	30
2. Rheumatic symptoms	35
3. Intestinal disorders	8
4. Pulmonary disorders	2

Criteria for diagnosis are:

1. Symmetrical weakness of the limb girdle muscles and anterior neck flexors.

2. Muscle biopsy showing necrosis of Type I and II fibres.

3. Elevation in serum of skeletal-muscle enzymes, particularly creatine phosphokinase (CPK).

4. Electromyographic changes – triad of short, small polyphasic motor units, fibrillations, positive sharp waves and insertional irritability and bizarre, high frequency repetitive discharges.

5. Dermatological features.

Except for childhood dermatomyositis, these conditions may appear at any time in life but are found more commonly in the mid-adult age group (40–50) with a predilection to women in a ratio of 3 : 1.

Muscle involvement

The common feature is muscle weakness due to diffuse inflammation of striated muscle. The changes observed on muscle biopsy are those of degeneration of muscle fibres, regeneration, infiltrates of chronic inflammatory cells, phagocytosis, interstitial fibrosis and variations in the cross sectional diameter of adjacent muscle fibres. It is important to note that regeneration is occurring at the same time as degeneration and it is probably this regeneration of muscle fibres that contributes to the return of muscle function in the recovery phase.

Brooke and Kaplan [5] in a study of 18 patients with polymyositis found marked variability of muscle fibre size on biopsy and there was atrophy of all fibre types.

The weakness is proximal and symmetrical and may be profound or so mild as to require considerable skill to detect. Muscle atrophy is only seen much later in the disease.

PURE POLYMYOSITIS

The disease may present as acute, chronic or sub-acute and typically the course of the disease is marked by periods of remission and exacerbation.

In the patient with acute disease, oedema of the skin over the affected muscles may be seen and the muscles are swollen and tender (Fig. 11.1).

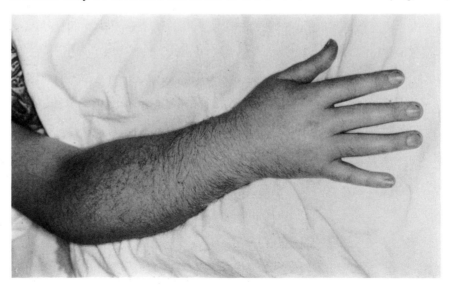

Fig. 11.1. Subcutaneous swelling of the forearm in a patient with polymyositis.

Joint pain is not a significant finding and, when it exists, is transitory and not a true arthralgia. As the oedema resolves, muscle atrophy is apparent with symmetrical weakness occurring in the muscles of the pelvic and shoulder girdles. The quadriceps and neck flexor muscles are then involved and ultimately more distal muscle groups. The muscles of respiration, swallowing and phonation may also be affected in severe disease, with the resultant risk of inhalation pneumonia.

By contrast, the patient who presents with sub-acute disease may simply describe increasing difficulty in functional activities such as climbing stairs, getting up from a chair or combing the hair, occurring over a period of many weeks or even months. The disease may not progress further or may remain static for long periods before progressing to involve other groups so that the patient becomes unable to sit up, turn in bed or walk.

In mild, chronic forms of polymyositis the muscle weakness may be so slight that the patient is unaware of the involvement and cursory examination will not reveal weakness to any but the skilled examiner.

Although the disease is essentially one of degeneration of striated muscle fibres, rarely there is also involvement of smooth muscle.

Polymyositis with other connective tissue disorders or rash

Patients placed in this diagnostic category are those who present with the clinical signs described above, but in addition exhibit features of other connective tissue diseases such as progressive systemic sclerosis. They may or may not show evidence of skin changes.

Joint symptoms may be present and are the manifestations of mild rheumatoid arthritis but the joint deformity and erosive changes of frank rheumatoid are not seen.

Severe connective tissue disease with incidental myositis

This group of patients is particularly difficult both to identify and to treat, because it is well established that in severe rheumatoid arthritis significant muscle wasting is found and, in addition, secondary steroid-induced myopathy may be present, further complicating the clinical picture. It has been conclusively demonstrated, by the use of electro-myography and muscle enzyme tests, that in a number of patients polymyositis co-exists with rheumatoid arthritis and other connective tissue disorders such as progressive systemic sclerosis, systemic lupus erythematosus and polyarteritis nodosa. It is important that these patients are identified because the use of steroids in this group of patients produces significant improvement.

Physiotherapy for the patient with polymyositis is discussed at the end of this chapter since the aims and objectives are similar for the whole group.

ADULT DERMATOMYOSITIS WITHOUT MALIGNANCY

Clinical features

The clinical features of dermatomyositis in adults are as those of polymyositis outlined previously, but in addition there are marked skin changes. Typically these skin manifestations are found over the face, neck, upper arms and upper trunk, although they may be found more extensively over the body, hand and lower limbs. The skin becomes characteristically erythematous and scaly and, later in the disease, atrophic. The skin changes over the hands, arms and legs more commonly occur over the extensor surfaces and are more scaly and atrophic; these are the 'collodion patches'.

The muscle weakness tends to be more severe and these patients often have more joint symptoms.

ADULT DERMATOMYOSITIS WITH MALIGNANCY

The strong association between dermatomyositis and malignancy has been established over many decades but the reason for it is unknown. The incidence of malignancy with dermatomyositis has been put at five to seven times that of the general population [6]. It has been suggested that improvement in the dermatomyositis follows treatment of the tumour [7].

CHILDHOOD DERMATOMYOSITIS

This is a distinct and well defined disorder and is probably due to an underlying angiopathy. Unlike adult dermatomyositis there is no association with malignancy but there is a higher incidence of joint involvement. There is considerable variability in the degree of rash or skin changes seen.

Clinical features

Muscle weakness is always present and is usually proximal and symmetrical, often starting in the pelvic girdle progressing to the thighs and upper shoulder girdle. The onset of the disease, which may occur at any age, is often insidious and frequently the first complaint is one of general malaise with a low grade fever. There may be pain and tenderness of muscles and occasionally subcutaneous oedema. The erythematous skin rash is typically seen over the malar area of the face but may be more widespread occurring over the extensor aspects of the arms and legs. There is usually a violaceous discoloration of the upper eyelids.

The combinations of muscle weakness, skin changes and general malaise seen are infinite.

Involvement of the respiratory muscles is seen more commonly in the younger age groups and indeed respiratory distress has been reported as the first major sign, probably due to involvement of the lung parenchyma [8].

The course of the disease is unpredictable and varied, with periods of remission punctuated by acute exacerbation.

In the chronic stage the child often presents with contractures at hips, knees, shoulders and ankles (Fig. 11.2a). The contractures are primarily due to the replacement of muscle fibre by fibrous tissue during the healing process but in childhood dermatomyositis the deposition of calcium in the interstitial tissues of muscle itself or in the subcutaneous tissues, seen more rarely in adult forms, is marked and may cause further disability (Fig. 11.2b). Nodules of calcium may even extrude through perforations in the skin. The incidence of calcinosis is variously recorded as occurring in 50–60% of cases.

Other systems that may be involved in childhood dermatomyositis are the reticuloendothelial, cardiovascular and gastrointestinal systems.

Typically the child has a waddling gait due to loss of power in the hip abductors and may be walking on the toes if contractures at the ankle are present. On examination there will be a true Trendelenberg sign. Changes seen in the muscle biopsy will be those of myopathy. It is this combination of findings that has caused some patients to be erroneously diagnosed as having limb girdle dystrophy.

Although the characteristic involvement described in the literature is in the proximal groups, clinical observation reveals that there is often a patchy weakness of more distal groups as well.

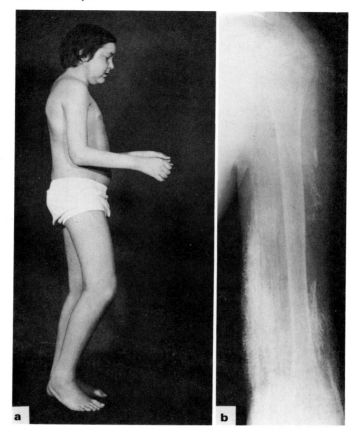

Fig. 11.2. (a) Fifteen year old boy with four year history of dermatomyositis. Note contractures at ankle, knee, hips, elbows and shoulders. (b) Radiograph of left humerus demonstrating calcinosis.

Course and prognosis

This is extremely variable and unpredictable. Exhaustive reviews of published series [9] indicate that approximately one-third died, one-third recovered completely or had only minimal signs and one-third were crippled to a severe or moderate degree.

TREATMENT OF POLYMYOSITIS AND DERMATOMYOSITIS

Drugs

Corticosteroids are used effectively in these conditions. The best dosage and drug regime is the subject of much investigation and controversy.

Immunosuppressive drugs such as methotrexate are also used but with caution and are reserved for those patients who have not responded to steroid therapy.

Rest

In the acute stage of the disease bed rest is indicated and attention to the prevention of contractures is essential. The bed should be firm and pillows should be carefully placed to prevent contractures developing at elbows and hips; the strategic placement of pillows will also maintain good head and neck posture. These patients have a typical inability to move and fracture boards placed beneath the mattress will provide a firmer platform for movement. The use of rest splints for the knee and ankle may be indicated.

Physiotherapy

AIMS

1. To prevent contractures
2. To maintain optimum function
3. To maintain adequate ventilation
4. To improve muscle power
5. To provide accurate assessment of muscle power of selected muscle groups for the purpose of monitoring drug therapy

METHODS

The general methods by which these aims are achieved are found in Chapters 2 and 4.

Maintenance of adequate ventilation

In the adult form of the disease respiration is rarely compromised but respiratory distress may be seen in the acute uncontrolled stage of disease; it is this small group of patients who may ultimately need assisted ventilation.

In childhood dermatomyositis, respiratory involvement is more common and aspiration pneumonia is sometimes seen in the younger age groups; attention to postural drainage and breathing exercises is indicated. For the detailed management of patients requiring ventilation and chest physiotherapy the reader should refer to an appropriate text [10].

EXERCISE

In both the adult and childhood forms of this disease, when the condition is so acute that the patient is on bed rest, exercise is confined to simple postural correction and static exercises for the hip and knee extensors, scapular retractors and gentle active assisted movements of the shoulder.

In the recovery period, for those patients who have been bed bound, exercise regimes are more rigorous and resisted exercises are used. We have found techniques of proprioceptive neuromuscular facilitation to be most beneficial in both strengthening muscle and regaining range of motion. Emphasis is again on the trunk musculature and resisted mat work is most helpful. Treatment in the prone position is used to facilitate neck flexors and promotes use of the stabilisers.

On discharge from hospital the patient is given a home programme of exercises with emphasis on the limb girdle muscles.

The majority of patients do not require hospitalisation and are well maintained on a home programme. A scheme of progressive resisted exercise is used and general activities are encouraged.

The collection of accurate serial measurements for monitoring progression of the disease and the effect of drug therapy require special mention (Fig. 11.3). Two indices are normally chosen, e.g. muscle power and functional level; details of this method of assessment are found in Chapter 3.

For the purpose of monitoring the effect of drug therapy it is sufficient to measure the muscle power of two groups. The quadriceps and shoulder abductors are commonly chosen, and are serially measured using standardised positions. The Hammersmith myometer is particularly useful for this purpose.

Functional level

Walking time over a measured distance is a convenient method.

Splinting for the correction of deformity

A word of caution is perhaps necessary on the use of splints, because of the presence of calcinosis. In the unfortunate circumstances that the patient is referred to physiotherapy relatively late in the course of the disease and marked calcification is already present, or where drug therapy has not controlled the disease process, X-rays must be taken before any attempt is made to correct the deformity. Serial plasters for the correction of deformity can only be used where the deformity is the result of fibrous tissue formation and calcinosis is not the limiting factor.

Case history

Mrs R. Age 31 years. (See Table 11.2 and Fig. 11.3)
February 1977
Developed pain and swelling of the distal interphalangeal and proximal interphalangeal joints both hands.
June 1977
Both wrists affected, bleeding of cuticles and erythematous rash over knuckles.

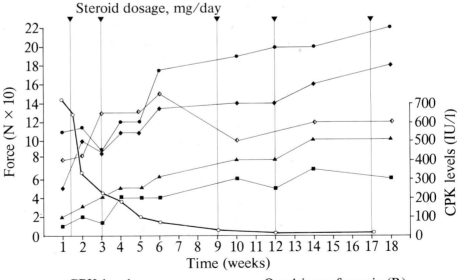

Fig. 11.3. The relationship of force output of selected muscle groups to steroid dosage and the level of circulating muscle enzymes in a patient (Mrs R.) with dermatomyositis.

○ CPK levels
• Foot dorsiflexors (R)
◇ Hip flexors (R)

• Quadriceps femoris (R)
▲ Shoulder abductors (R)
■ Neck flexors

Table 11.2.

PHYSIOTHERAPY DEPARTMENT

Example of measurements of patient with adult dermatomyositis (Mrs R.)

Name: Mrs R.
Address:
Time: 9.00 a.m.
In-patient: X
Out-patient:
Muscle Function Study: No

Case Note No:
Age: 31 years
Height: 160 cms
Weight: 53.6 kg
Dominant Hand: Right
Physiotherapy Treatment:
Ward Class
Name of Dr:
Diagnosis: Dermatomyositis

Active Resisted Exercises, concentrating on trunk, and bilateral limb patterns.

Date 25.4.78

Muscle Strength (newtons × 10)	Agst Grav	Best Effort	Right	Best Effort	Best Effort	Left	Best Effort	Best Effort
Foot D/F	8.0	9.0	9.0	9.0	11.0	7.0	7.0	11.0
Quadriceps	9.0	9.5	9.0	9.5	7.0	8.0	7.5	8.0
Knee flexion								
Hip flexion	12.0	12.0	13.0	13.0	9.0	10.0	10.5	10.5
Hip abduction								
Hip extension								
Shoulder abduction	4.0	3.5	3.0	4.0	3.0	4.0	3.0	4.0
Elbow flexion	4.5	3.5		4.5	4.0	4.0		4.0
Elbow extension	2.0	3.5		3.5	2.5	2.0		2.0
Wrist extension	2.0	2.5	4.0	4.0	2.0	2.0	3.5	3.5
Neck flexion	1.0	1.5		1.5	2.0	2.0		

Grip strength (mm Hg) 158   9.5
Walk time (secs)
P/T Sig.   SC

Comments: Managing stairs more easily.
Grip strengths have improved.
To remain on 30 mg Prednisilone.

October 1977
Complained of painful muscles and difficulty in moving.
April 1978
Admitted to hospital for further investigations.

> *Findings.* Difficulty in walking
> Rising from chair
> Dressing
> Combing hair

> *Muscle biopsy.* Confirmed diagnosis of active dermatomyositis with vasculitis.

> *Drug therapy.* Systemic steroids: Prednisone 40 mg/day reduced to 30 mg/day after 10 days.

> *Physiotherapy.* Ward class – active free exercise. Manually resisted exercises to strengthen.

It was possible to monitor the improvement of strength of selected muscle groups using a hand held myometer and to plot these graphically with the level of steroid dosage and the level of circulating muscle enzymes (see Fig. 11.3).

Mrs R. was discharged home after six weeks and was maintained on a home programme, only attending the department for revision of the programme.

September 1978
Fully mobile and managing well.
October 1978
Became pregnant – treatment stopped.

Case history

Fifteen year old schoolboy (Mr P.) diagnosed as having dermatomyositis. (See Fig. 11.2a, b and Table 11.3.)
April 1976
Presented with ten month history of rash and muscle stiffness. Treated with daily prednisolone.
November 1976
Referred to Hammersmith for assessment and drug management. Prednisolone reduced to alternate days.
March 1977
Commenced regular physiotherapy and hydrotherapy at local hospital because muscular weakness had increased and functional impairment

was marked, unable to rise from toilet or floor unaided. Prednisolone increased.

April 1977

Tender over left 4th rib – probable crack fracture from steroid-induced osteoporosis.

June 1977

Azathioprine started in addition to steroids. Continued to deteriorate, just able to lift his head and limbs against gravity because of severe muscle weakness and atrophy. Walking time increased. Admitted to hospital for therapy.

July 1977

Much improved.

August 1977

Steroids reduced.

Azathioprine continued.

Patient complaining of lumbar ache – X-rays showed minimal osteoporosis.

February 1978

Admitted to hospital for one week because of azathioprine-induced diarrhoea.

Table 11.3. Serial measurements of patient with childhood dermatomyositis (Mr P.).

	Right			Left		
	12.2.77	17.6.77	28.2.78	12.2.77	17.6.77	28.2.78
Muscle strength (Newtons × 10)						
Muscle group						
Foot D'F	12	5.5	15	11	7.5	15
Quadriceps	15	4.5	off scale	13	4.5	off scale
Knee flexion	12	6	7	12	5.5	6.5
Hip flexion	4	0	6.5	9	0	8
Hip abduction	9	5	6.5	5	6	9
Hip extension	6	0	8.5	7	0	8.5
Shoulder abduction	3	0	6.5	4.5	0	6
Wrist extension	4	2	7	4	2	5
Neck flexion	3	3	4.5			
Contractures (Angular degrees)						
Elbow F.D.	—	15	20	—	10	20
Hip F.D.	—	0	8	—	0	10
Knee F.D.	35	0	8	35	0	0
Shoulder abduction	0	0	0	0	0	0
Oxford grading (% total MRC)	74	54.7	78			

November 1978

Admitted to hospital for two weeks because of a relapse.

May 1979

Now attending school three full days a week.

Physiotherapy has continued on an out-patient basis since March 1977 and has consisted of active resisted exercises to improve muscle power and maintain mobility and range of motion. Splints for the lower extremities have also been used in an attempt to prevent deformity. Serial measurements have been made and are as shown in Table 11.3. Unfortunately, unremitting calcinosis has occurred and has now compromised range of motion in both upper and lower extremities.

REFERENCES

[1] WALTON J. N. & ADAMS R. D. (1958) *Polymyositis*. Livingstone, Edinburgh.

[2] ROSE A. L. & WALTON J. N. (1966) Polymyositis: a survey of 89 cases with particular reference to treatment and prognosis. *Brain*, **89**, 747–768.

[3] PEARSON C. M. (1966) Polymyositis. *Annual Review of Medicine*, **17**, 63–82.

[4] BARWICK D. D. & WALTON J. N. (1963) Polymyositis. *American Journal of Medicine*, **35**, 646–660.

[5] BROOKE M. H. & KAPLAN H. (1972) Muscle pathology in rheumatoid arthritis, polymyalgia rheumatica and polymyositis. *Archives of Pathology*, **94**, 101–118.

[6] BARNES B. E. (1976) Dermatomyositis and malignancy. A review of the literature. *Annals of Internal Medicine*, **84**, 68–76.

[7] ARUNDELL F. D., WILKINSON R. D. & HASERICK J. R. (1960) Dermatomyositis and malignant neoplasms in adults. *Archives of Dermatology*, **82**, 772.

[8] DUBOWITZ L. M. S. & DUBOWITZ V. (1964) Acute dermatomyositis presenting with pulmonary manifestations. *Archives of Disease in Childhood*, **39**, 293–296.

[9] MEDSGER T. A. JR., ROBINSON H. & MASI A. T. (1971) Factors affecting survivorship in polymyositis. *Arthritis and Rheumatism*, **14**, 249–258.

[10] GASKELL D. V. & WEBBER B. A. (1977) *The Brompton Hospital Guide to Chest Physiotherapy*. 3rd Ed. Blackwell, Oxford.

12 Progressive Systemic Sclerosis (Scleroderma)

This disease is more frequently called scleroderma because of the characteristic changes seen in the skin of afflicted patients but the manifestations of the disease are widespread and serious. The onset of the disease is usually between 20–50 years of age and women are affected more than men in a ratio of 4:1, there is also a greater incidence in Negroes than in Caucasians.

AETIOLOGY

The aetiology of the disease remains unknown and there is no clear evidence of familial incidence. The increased incidence of the disease amongst certain groups, e.g. coal miners, has led some investigators to look at environmental factors for causal agents. The most active investigations are by those workers looking at collagen synthesis, the role of capillary changes and immunological aspects of the disease.

PATHOLOGY

Although this systemic disease may ultimately affect many of the body's organs, the changes of fibrosis, vascular insufficiency and ischaemic atrophy are common to all the structures involved.

In the early skin stages there is oedema, with over-production of collagen and abnormalities of mucopolysaccharides. It is the increased dermal collagen and the reduction in elasticity which gives rise to the characteristic thickening and immobility.

Fibrosis may also occur in the cardiac muscle, oesophagus and small gut in the late stages of the disease there is pulmonary involvement.

The changes seen in the kidneys and liver are the result of fibrinoid changes in the artery and arteriole walls.

CLINICAL FEATURES

The clinical pattern of progressive systemic sclerosis varies widely but about 80% develop *Raynaud's phenomenon* and this may herald the other overt signs of the disease by many months or even years.

Raynaud's phenomenon is characterised by hypersensitivity to cold resulting from small artery spasm, the digits of the patient often becoming cyanosed and, on re-heating, becoming swollen, painful and dusky red in appearance (Fig. 12.1). The patient often develops small intractable ulcers on the finger tips.

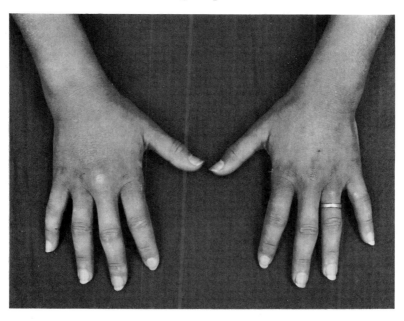

Fig. 12.1. Patient with early scleroderma. Note mottled and swollen appearance of fingers, also small ulcer over the metacarpophalangeal joints.

Skin

The earliest change is oedema and in the hands this will result in tense swollen fingers but as the disease progresses there is thickening and tethering of the skin spreading proximally to involve upper limbs, face, trunk and lower limbs. The skin becomes shiny, taut and hairless, with loss of sweating. In the fingers these changes make the digit appear to taper with atrophy of the pulp, hence the word sclerodactyly is used. The facial appearance is changed, the skin around the nose and mouth becoming taut, with radial furrowing around the mouth. There may also be changes in skin pigmentation.

CALCINOSIS

This occurs in the skin and subcutaneous tissues, usually restricted to the fingers but occasionally more widespread (Fig. 12.2). Sometimes calcific material is extruded through the small ulcers that develop on the finger tips.

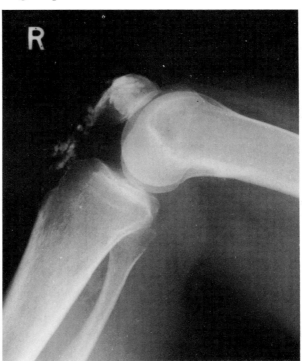

Fig. 12.2. Radiograph of right knee of patient with scleroderma showing calcinosis of patella tendon.

Muscles and joints

Muscle weakness is evident in this condition and may in the late stages be severe. The proximal muscles, particularly those of the shoulder girdle and neck, are most commonly affected, although more distal groups may also be involved. Inflammatory myositis is seen in approximately one-third of patients. In the past, relatively little attention has been given to the myopathic features of this disease but recent work has highlighted the importance of these changes [1].

The joint involvement seen in progressive systemic sclerosis is mainly confined to the small joints of the hands but may occasionally affect other joints. Unlike rheumatoid arthritis, erosive changes do not usually occur, but in the early stages of the disease the polyarthritis, seen in approximately one-third of patients, is just as troublesome and incapacitating.

The joint contractures seen are due to thickening and tethering of the skin, together with fibrosis of the joint capsule and tendon sheaths (Fig. 12.3).

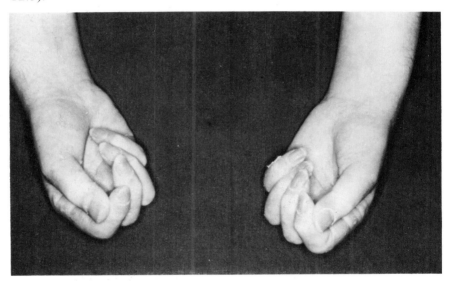

Fig. 12.3. Advanced contractures in patient with scleroderma.

Gastrointestinal tract

1. Microstomia, the narrowed puckered mouth, leads to difficulties with eating, which is further hampered by decreased parotid secretions.

2. Dysphagia occurs as a result of loss of mobility of the oesophagus.

3. Steatorrhoea, malabsorption and weight loss all occur as mobility of the gut and small bowel are reduced.

The lungs

Pulmonary involvement is seen in about 30% of patients but is often asymptomatic. The changes are those of restrictive lung disease and pulmonary function tests may show a reduced diffusing capacity.

Occasionally aspiration pneumonia occurs secondary to reflux oesophagitis.

The heart

Cardiomyopathy and intractable heart failure occur in 50% of patients.

The combined effect of heart and lung involvement produces dyspnoea of effort.

Kidney

Hypertension occurs with the involvement of the kidneys late in the disease and is life threatening.

Liver

It has only recently been recognised that the disease process affects the liver, producing portal hypertension and biliary cirrhosis.

LABORATORY TESTS

Muscle enzyme levels – often unchanged
ESR – moderately raised
Serum globulins – moderately raised
Immunological abnormalities are common but non-specific
Rheumatoid factor is positive in approximately 40%

TREATMENT

No really effective treatment has yet been discovered.

Drugs

Corticosteroids – limited use because of the danger of producing hypertension

Collagen production inhibitors, e.g. D-penicillamine
Immunosuppressors
Vasodilators – these have doubtful value.

Physiotherapy

Physiotherapy in progressive systemic sclerosis is often unrewarding, the disease progressing in a relentless way, but even small improvements are meaningful to the patient and diligent care can prevent the early contractures and loss of function seen in the untreated case.

AIMS OF PHYSIOTHERAPY

1. To prevent contractures and loss of mobility
2. To preserve muscle power
3. To educate the patient

METHODS

Exercise
Passive stretching
Massage
Splinting

Exercise, using techniques of proprioceptive neuromuscular facilitation, is directed at strengthening the muscles of the neck, shoulder girdle and upper limbs. The same techniques are particularly helpful in these patients to improve chest wall mobility and improve ventilation, in preference to the more orthodox breathing exercises.

Passive stretching of the small joints of the hand and wrist, preceded by hot paraffin wax baths, may be helpful in the early stages of the disease. Care must be taken when using wax baths because of the vascular component of the disease and the skin should be thoroughly inspected for any signs of ulceration or impending ulceration.

Massage. The most effective method of both preventing and treating contractures is connective tissue massage and details of this are found in other texts [2].

Lanolin massage using deep kneading is helpful in preserving the integrity of the skin of the hands, in particular around the nailbeds, and over the proximal interphalangeal, interphalangeal and metacarpophalangeal joints.

Splintage. In the early stage of the disease rest splints may be of some value to prevent contractures in the hand and wrist. These splints must be very carefully fitted to avoid further compromising the circulation and to avoid pressure areas. When such splints are used it is essential that they are frequently reviewed.

Stretch plasters are used to correct deformities of the metacarpophalangeal, interphalangeal and proximal interphalangeal joints that result from skin and tendon tethering. The plasters are changed at 2–3 day intervals. Use of stretch plasters is combined with active exercises.

Cervical collars are sometimes used in the late stages of the disease when there is marked involvement of the neck muscles, particularly the posterior group.

PATIENT EDUCATION

When Raynaud's phenomenon is present, the patient is advised about the use of warm gloves, heated gloves and other protective clothing.

Advice on skin care, the avoidance of minor trauma, and passive stretching is essential and the patient should be encouraged to carry out a home programme of exercises.

PROGNOSIS

Progressive systemic sclerosis is a multi-system life threatening disease and most patients will die from it within ten years of onset. The course of the disease is unpredictable and the length of survival is determined by the degree and progression of the disease within the kidneys, lungs and gastrointestinal tract.

Case history

Miss C., aged 26 years, was well until 1977. (See Table 12.1.)
December 1977
During a very cold spell she developed severe Raynaud's phenomenon.

Table 12.1. Serial measurements of patient (Miss C.) with progressive systemic sclerosis.

Assessment right hand	26.6.78	24.7.78	26.8.78	2.10.78	9.1.79	1.5.79
Grip strength (mmHg)	176	202	154	110	133	123
Flexion deficit (cm)						
1st wrist crease						
Index finger	5.50	5.25	6.25	5.0	5.25	5.1
Third finger	5.00	3.75	5.25	4.5	6.00	5.3
Ring finger	4.25	2.25	4.25	3.5	4.50	4.5
Little finger	5.00	4.25	5.75	3.0	3.50	3.5
Extension (cm)						
1st wrist crease						
Index finger	—	—	—	11.2	15.00	14.0
Third finger	—	—	—	9.5	14.50	14.0
Ring finger	—	—	—	7.0	14.00	13.6
Little finger	—	—	—	6.5	12.00	12.0
Chest expansion (cm)	4.00	5.00	6.00	4.0	7.00	7.0
Maximum mouth open (cm)	3.50	4.00	4.50	4.0	4.50	4.0

February 1978
She developed a generalised arthralgia affecting her knees, ankles, metatarsophalangeal joints, shoulders, elbows, wrists and hands. Home programme of maintenance exercise.

May 1978
Admitted to hospital for full investigation. Complaining of morning stiffness, persistent pain and stiffness of her hands, difficulty in swallowing and great difficulty in moving after resting. On examination she had tight skin over fingers and wrist with tendon contractures. Painful bilateral knee effusions, right more than left. Facial tightness with difficulty in opening her mouth and a stooping posture.

Physiotherapy. Active exercises in ward class. Massage with lanolin and resting splints for her hands.

September 1978
Re-admitted with a flare of polyarthralgia and complaining of pleuritic type chest pains. She commented on the progression of skin changes and she had increased contractures of her hands.

Physiotherapy. Active exercises in ward class, wax baths and massage. Careful splinting was undertaken in an attempt to ease the pain and prevent further development and progression of contractures.

April 1979
Admitted for re-assessment. She was generally improved but had persistent contractures of her fingers and considerable skin thickening which extended to her forearms.

REFERENCES

[1] MEDSGER T. A. JR., RODNAN G. P., MOOSSY J. & VESTOR J. W. (1968) Skeletal muscle involvement in progressive systemic sclerosis (scleroderma). *Arthritis and Rheumatism*, **11,** 554–568.

[2] EBNER M. (1975) *Connective Tissue Massage*, pp. 143–149. R. E. Krieger, Huntingdon, New York.

13 Miscellaneous Rheumatological Diseases

PSORIATIC ARTHROPATHY

This is one of the sero-negative group of diseases, and as its name suggests is an arthropathy classically associated with psoriasis. It should not be confused with rheumatoid disease with which there may be incidental psoriasis.

Pattern of joint involvement

Characteristically the distal interphalangeal joints of the fingers, the interphalangeal joints of the toes and the interphalangeal joint of the thumb are affected. The spine and sacroiliac joints may also be involved, as indeed may other peripheral joints, but less frequently and in unpredictable patterns. The pattern of joint involvement is significant in differential diagnosis since the onset of psoriasis does not always precede joint involvement.

Natural history

The arthropathy once present tends to follow a course which is either benign or severe and aggressive, unlike rheumatoid arthritis which follows an erratic but chronic course over many years.

The patient commonly presents with a history of psoriasis which is in remission at the onset of joint involvement. The joint is hot and swollen and there is marked evidence of synovial disease. As the disease progresses erosive changes occur with loss of bone. In the most severe form of the disease, joint destruction with absorption of bone and consequent deformity with loss of function occurs. Those patients who exhibit this severe destructive form of the disease are said to have 'arthritis mutilans'.

Pathology

The pathological changes seen in the joints are similar to those seen in rheumatoid arthritis but the systemic features of rheumatoid disease are not found in psoriatic arthropathy. This is significant from the physiotherapist's viewpoint (Table 13.1).

Table 13.1. Comparison of changes seen in rheumatoid arthritis and psoriatic arthropathy.

	Rheumatoid arthritis	Psoriatic arthropathy
Typical joint involvement	MCP Wrist	DIP
Nodules	Yes	No
Blood tests		
Rh factor	Yes	No
ESR	Yes	No
Other systems		
Muscle	Yes	No
Tendon	Yes	No
Lung	Yes	No
Psoriasis	Occasional	Always
Radiological changes	Erosions	Yes
	Osteoporosis	Yes
	Periosteal new bone	+ +

Physiotherapy

In the less severe form minimal treatment is required and is primarily directed toward joint protection and maintenance of function. The methods of achieving these are as discussed in Chapters 2 and 4. Since the gross muscle and tendon involvement of rheumatoid arthritis is not seen, there is not such a demand for intensive rehabilitation.

In arthritis mutilans it is the severe loss of bone that causes the gross deformity and dysfunction. Attempts to prevent deformity by such methods as splinting are fruitless in this condition and the physiotherapist simply attempts to maintain function by a home programme of exercises. The occupational therapist may have a significant role in the provision of aids and adaptations.

REITER'S DISEASE

This is a sero-negative polyarticular arthropathy of unknown cause with a predilection for males in the third and fourth decades.

The joint involvement is characteristically limited to the lower extremities and spine and typically begins in the knees, ankles and mid-tarsal joints. There is a marked tendency to inflammation of the tendon sheaths and fascia, particularly of the tendo-achilles and plantar fascia.

The disease is associated with non-gonococcal infection of the genital tract, dysentery or non-specific diarrhoea.

In many cases the disease is self limiting and only a small percentage suffer recurrent attacks, when they develop a clinical picture which is similar to that of ankylosing spondylitis. Urethritis, prostatitis, conjunctivitis and skin and mucosal lesions are frequently seen in association with the disease.

Physiotherapy

ACUTE STAGE

The joint or joints affected should be treated as for any other acute inflammatory arthropathy but immobilisation or splinting is avoided because there is an increased tendency to develop stiffness and muscle wasting. The methods used are gentle, free active exercise to maintain range of movement, isometric strengthening exercises and ice for the relief of pain.

The use of walking aids is indicated to relieve pain in weight bearing joints.

Where the classical achilles tendinitis or plantar fasciitis occur ultrasound may be beneficial. Temporary modification of footwear may be helpful.

CHRONIC STAGE

In these patients who suffer recurrent attacks and eventually develop spondylitis, physiotherapy is as outlined for ankylosing spondylitis.

JACCOUD'S SYNDROME

This is a rare variety of chronic sero-negative arthritis characterised by fibrous changes in joint capsules and tendons leading to deformities resembling rheumatoid arthritis. Unlike rheumatoid the erythrocyte sedimentation rate is not elevated.

Physiotherapy

Physiotherapy consists mainly of endeavours to prevent deformity by splinting and exercises.

TIETZE'S SYNDROME

This involves the costo-chondral joints causing anterior chest pain which may radiate into the lateral chest wall.

Ultrasound is often helpful in reducing the swelling and tenderness.

POLYARTERITIS NODOSA

This is a generalised connective tissue disorder, affecting males more than females, in which there is involvement of all three layers of the walls of the small and medium sized arteries by an acute inflammatory process which leads ultimately to necrosis.

Clinical features

The disease may start anywhere in the body and more than one system may be compromised, so that the patient may present with:

1. Fever and arthralgia
2. Renal disease
3. Pulmonary disease
4. Neurological lesions
5. Cardiovascular lesions
6. Musculoskeletal involvement

Treatment

Drugs: Corticosteroids.

Physiotherapy: This is indicated where the patient presents with musculoskeletal involvement or neurological lesions. The physical management is then similar to that for rheumatoid arthritis with arteritis but deformity is rare.

SJØGREN'S SYNDROME

This is one of the connective tissue diseases and affects females to males in a ratio of 9:1. It is by definition a disease in which there is poly-arthritis of the rheumatoid type associated with dryness of the eyes and mouth.

It is an autoimmune disease presenting with widespread and variable clinical manifestations. It may affect:

Ear, nose, throat
Liver
Genito-urinary tract
Nervous system
Respiratory system
Vascular system

Physiotherapy

The physiotherapy is as described for rheumatoid arthritis but where the upper respiratory tract is affected recurrent chest infections may require more attention to breathing exercises. Patients with this disease undergoing surgery will need more treatment postoperatively and attention to adequate humidification.

14 Osteoarthrosis

The inclusion of a short chapter on osteoarthrosis in this text, concerned as it is with the rheumatological diseases, may seem strange. There are two reasons for its inclusion, firstly that secondary osteoarthrosis may occur as a result of rheumatoid arthritis (Fig. 14.1), and secondly that the physiotherapist working in a rheumatology clinic may see many cases of osteoarthrosis. The subject of degenerative joint disease (osteoarthrosis) has been covered in much larger texts and physiotherapy journals, so that here only a brief outline of the pathology and clinical features is given. Emphasis is placed on the differences in the physiotherapy management between osteoarthrosis and the rheumatological disorders.

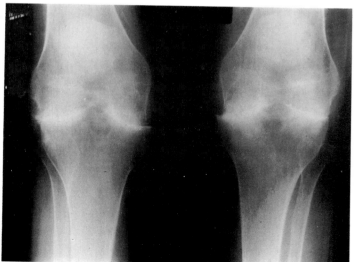

Fig. 14.1. Radiograph showing secondary degenerative changes in knees of patient with rheumatoid arthritis.

Primary osteoarthrosis. Degenerative changes occur in an otherwise normal joint. It occurs mainly in women and is characterised by Heberden's nodes and bony enlargement of the first metacarpophalangeal joint. Early in the disease there is spontaneous pain, which is worse after exercise and at night, but morning stiffness is not a feature of the disease. The pain remits as cartilage and ligaments become ossified.

Secondary osteoarthrosis. The changes are directly attributable to a cause, for example changes in the geometry or physical properties of the joint.

AETIOLOGY

These may be summarised as:

Genetic factors
Metabolic factors
Endocrine abnormalities
Inflammatory arthropathies
Anatomical abnormalities
Trauma
Neuropathic causes

PATHOLOGY

The primary pathological change seen in osteoarthrosis occurs in the hyaline cartilage covering the articular surfaces of bone. The cartilage of a normal joint serves to provide a smooth, frictionless and compressible surface on which movement can occur. In degenerative joint disease the cartilage becomes softened and there is separation of the superficial fibres. Flakes of cartilage then break away into the synovial fluid; clinically this may present as a mild synovitis.

Cartilage has no direct blood supply and obtains its nutrition from the synovial fluid, the normal movement of the joint ensuring adequate circulation over the entire surface. The cartilage once damaged does not regenerate because of the nature of the blood supply.

The second stage in osteoarthrosis is new bone formation which may be seen as osteophyte formation at the joint margin, the subchondral bone also becoming thickened. The altered stresses and strains on the bone produce micro-fractures and later cystic changes are seen. As the joint continues to be used the cartilage over the joint surface becomes increasingly roughened and ultimately the bone is exposed. This bone responds initially by becoming eburnated but later disintegrates and collapses under the strain.

CLINICAL FEATURES

The main features are pain in the region of the joint, progressive loss of joint range and deformity. The pain of osteoarthritis varies from a mild ache to severe pain, sometimes sufficient to cause disturbed sleep patterns, the mechanism of which is not fully understood. The progression of the disease and the number of joints involved is variable, although commonly only one joint is affected, and relates to the aetiological factors previously listed. Unlike rheumatoid arthritis, it is not a systemic disease and where structures other than those of the joint are affected it is the direct result of mechanical derangement.

Factors which affect the course and progression of the disease are age, weight and occupation.

The deformity seen in osteoarthrosis is the product of altered joint geometry, but the joint instability, so frequently seen in rheumatoid

Table 14.1. Comparison of laboratory findings and radiological changes.

	Osteoarthrosis	Rheumatoid arthritis
Blood tests		
ESR	Normal	Elevated
Rh. factor	Absent	Present
LE cell count	Negative	Positive in 10% of patients
Synovial fluid	Clear	More opaque
	Low cell count	Increased cell count
	Normal viscosity	Low viscosity
	Protein count slightly increased	Increased
X-ray changes		
Loss of joint space	Yes	Yes
Erosions	No	Yes
Osteophytes	Yes	No
Bone density	Sclerotic	Porotic
Cystic formation	Frequent	Occasional

disease, is rarely found. Muscle wasting is observed in chronic degenerative disease but is of the simple disuse atrophy type, there is no primary involvement of muscle.

Degenerative joint disease is more common in the major weight-bearing joints but may occur in the hand, elbow, shoulder and spine. The characteristic pattern and progression of joint involvement seen in the rheumatological disorders are not found.

TREATMENT

Drugs

Anti-inflammatory analgesics are used to control pain but are often less effective than in other situations.

Conservative measures

These include advice on dietary habits to prevent or reduce obesity, avoidance of occupational aggravation and advice on stress relieving postures during activities of daily living.

Surgery

In the late stages of the disease or where persistent pain is affecting the quality of life surgery may be undertaken (Figs. 14.2 and 14.3a, b).

Physiotherapy

AIMS

1. To prevent further strain or trauma on an affected joint
2. To improve muscle power
3. To improve nutrition of the cartilage by restoration of physiological movement

METHODS

1. Exercise
2. Patient education
3. Mobilisation
4. Provision of aids

Adjuncts: Ice and heat.

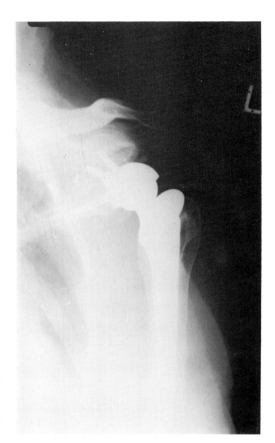

Fig. 14.2. Arthroplasty of left shoulder in patient with incapacitating pain and loss of function resulting from osteoarthrosis.

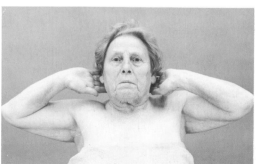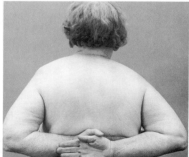

Fig. 14.3. Patient in Fig. 14.2, three years post-operatively, showing painless functional range of motion.

Exercise

Exercise in degenerative joint disease increases the strength of muscles acting over the affected joint and thereby improves the body's natural splinting mechanism to prevent further trauma or strain on the joint. In choosing the technique of exercise consideration is given to the position in which the exercise is performed and the excursion through which the movement is performed. Excessive range of motion or compression, as in weight bearing, will only serve to increase the trauma to the joint. Isometric exercises are used when the joint is painful and carefully graduated resistance exercises through controlled range are substituted as pain remits. Where exercise is used to gain range of motion, proprioceptive neuromuscular facilitation techniques of hold relax are most beneficial. In osteoarthrosis of the lumbo-sacral spine and lower limb, stabilising exercises for the lower trunk and walking re-education are essential.

Patient education

The physician, on making the diagnosis of osteoarthrosis, carefully explains to the patient the limitations that the disease may impose on occupation and leisure activities. The patient is reassured that it is not the crippling disease, rheumatoid arthritis; this is very important since the average lay person uses only the generalised term arthritis. The physiotherapist reinforces this view and gives careful and specific advice with regard to posture, amount of activity and rest.

As already stated where the lumbar spine or major joints of the lower limb are affected walking re-education is of paramount importance. The patient is discouraged from limping as this will only throw additional strain on to adjacent joints and joints of the opposite limb. Attention to footwear is vital and in the later stages of the disease, where deformity may produce limb length disparity, shoe raises are invaluable.

Mobilisation techniques

The acceptance and increasing use of techniques of mobilisation, together with more understanding of the method of nutrition of joint cartilage has significantly improved the contribution that physiotherapy can make in the treatment of degenerative joint disease. The reader is referred to the appropriate texts on this subject [1, 2].

Provision of aids

This is essentially the prescription of aids to mobility and in the late stages of the disease the use of calipers in the lower limb to prevent painful movement and trauma.

The earlier use of walking sticks is advocated in an attempt to prevent unwanted stress being placed on other joints and to preserve a mechanically more efficient walking pattern.

Use of adjuncts

It has been traditional through the years for patients with osteoarthrosis to be referred to physiotherapy departments and most referrals have included the request for heat. Relatively little investigative work has been undertaken on the effects of these treatments (short-wave diathermy, infra-red, etc.), partly because of the inherent difficulties in undertaking clinical trials. However, one study [3] reported that ice was found most beneficial in relieving pain in osteoarthrosis.

In summary, although osteoarthrosis results in joint dysfunction as rheumatoid arthritis does, it is not a multisystem disease and the muscle atrophy is less profound and of Type II fibre involvement from disuse. The aims and methods of physiotherapy reflect these differences emphasising exercise for the restoration of muscle strength for control and passive techniques for improved joint range.

REFERENCES
[1] MAITLAND G. D. (1977) *Peripheral Manipulation*. 2nd Ed. Butterworths, London.
[2] MAITLAND G. D. (1977) *Vertebral Manipulation*. 4th Ed. Butterworths, London.
[3] CLARKE G. R., WILLIS L. A., STENNER L. & NICHOLS P. J. R. (1974) Evaluation of physiotherapy in the treatment of osteoarthrosis of the knee. *Rheumatology and Rehabilitation*, **13,** 190–197.

15 Social Aspects

The physiotherapist treating patients with one of the rheumatological disorders must be aware of the social aspects and implications of the disease. It is not her fundamental role to attempt to act as counsellor or pseudo-medical social worker nor indeed should her medical colleagues attempt to use the skills of the physiotherapist as a psychological prop. It is essential, though, that she has sufficient understanding and knowledge of the emotional and social disruption that this group of diseases can cause, to recognise early and often disguised pleas for help by her patients. She is then able to make appropriate referrals to those properly trained in these aspects of management. Further, sympathetic understanding will enhance the patient's response to physical measures by improving compliance with treatment regimes.

It is a basic premise that an individual's emotional and psychological response to the effects of disease is as singular and personal as the response to any other major incident or experience in life. It is also essential that the patient feels that he or she has the right to choose and make decisions about treatment and this fact must be accepted by those concerned in rehabilitation. It is the physiotherapist's task to ensure that the patient understands the consequences of non-compliance with treatment programmes and so does not make decisions in ignorance but it is not her role to undermine the patient's active participation in decision making.

In order to comprehend the effect the disease may have on the individual, it is necessary to look at the various components and these may be summarised as social background, social disruption caused by the disease, the patient's psycho-social response to the disease and the effect of long term illness with threatened disablement.

The patient with one of the rheumatological disorders, on being told the diagnosis, immediately or gradually becomes aware of the effect that the disease may have on the structure and quality of life. Concern and doubts develop about the future role as housewife, mother, bread-winner, or head of household and the ability to live a full life both at work and at leisure. The patient is perturbed at the prospect of changed appearance because of deformity and the social stigma of being a cripple [1]. The trained therapist is aware that many of the fears are of little substance because with preventive measures, adequate treatment and the help from other agencies, disability can be minimised; but the patient does not know and maximum opportunity for the patient to discuss his/her fears at this early stage is essential. This is particularly important because in the early stages of the disease when there may not be obvious signs to the casual observer, other people are often not as understanding as the patient would wish. The patient's reaction at this time may be one of anxiety or reactive depression. As the disease continues the following responses may be seen: denial of the disease, hostility, with-drawal, dependency and acceptance of the disease. Sensitive help and understanding can prevent the patient becoming an emotional cripple and help to maintain psychological equilibrium. Regrettably there has developed an attitude by some clinicians that there is a 'rheumatoid psychology' or 'rheumatoid personality'. This hypothesis is often passed on to relatives and other members of the team caring for the patient, and yet there are few controlled trials to substantiate this theory. Indeed much of the work undertaken in this area would seem to indicate that the patient with one of the rheumatological disorders exhibits the same or similar responses as patients with other long term chronic diseases [2, 3, 4].

In the preceding chapters where the physiotherapy aims and objectives have been discussed there has been an emphasis on patient education. In helping the patient understand the disease, its manifestations and the physical management, the physiotherapist is also helping the patient achieve social and emotional stability and minimise the disruptive elements of the disease on these aspects of life. Although population studies demonstrate a high incidence of rheumatological disorders, the general public remains remarkably ill-informed and many patients and their relatives will be of the belief that a diagnosis of rheumatoid arthritis is synonymous with a wheelchair existence. The nature and erratic course of this group of diseases makes it essential that patients receive long term support. This does not mean that frequent hospital attendance is necessary, but regular follow-up will be. The physio-therapist treating such patients is wise to remember that they will be particularly sensitive to any sign of withdrawal or lack of commitment on the part of the therapist. The patient needs to feel as important and cared for in the quiescent stage as during an acute exacerbation. In a busy out-patient department it is often too easy to appear to reject or withdraw from the chronic and well-known patient in favour of the more acute orthopaedic patient.

Hostility, overt or disguised, may be the response to pain, fear or depression and an angry or sharp retort by the therapist will only entrench these feelings and may make the patient reject further help. Quiet but firm counselling and an attentive ear may help the patient understand the basis of his/her reaction.

The patient's feelings of guilt and anxiety at being a burden to the family [5] and concern over the disruption that impaired mobility may make on all aspects of family life may be helped by encouraging other members of the family to become involved in the treatment programme. In this way it is often possible for the physiotherapist to act as a catalyst in assisting other members of the family to seek counselling. The disease may effect employment opportunities with consequent financial strain and put stress on interpersonal relationships and marital harmony. If rehabilitation is to be complete, maximum help and support in all these aspects is needed.

The patient with chronic disabling disease may need help at different stages and of varying type. The physiotherapist must be aware of the contribution to be made by the medical social worker, disablement resettlement officer, marriage guidance, social service agencies and voluntary organisations and make appropriate referrals.

The provision of aids by the occupational therapist [6] is of great consequence because, in addition to making self care possible and so pre-serving independence, it will enable the patient to save physical energy. This means that he or she will have more energy to enjoy leisure activities and a full social life. It is essential, therefore, that close co-operation exists between the occupational therapist and the physiotherapist.

In summary then it may be said a failure on the part of either patient or therapist to recognise the psycho-social effects of the disease and an unwillingness to deal positively with these effects will present a barrier to management. The degree of success in coping socially will be tempered by external factors, namely economic and occupational and the availability of local community resources and legislation.

The erratic course of many rheumatological disorders and their ability to cause impairment of mobility and self care may cause varying degrees of disruption in the patient's social fabric. Therapy and physical management will be most effective where social aspects of the disease are treated positively and the patient's social assets emphasised.

REFERENCES

[1] GOFFMAN E. (1968) *Stigma: Notes on the Management of Spoiled Identity.* Penguin, Harmondsworth.
[2] SENESCU R. A. (1963) The development of emotional complications in the patient with cancer. *Journal of Chronic Diseases,* **16,** 813–832.
[3] VIGNOS P. J. JR., THOMPSON H. M., KATZ S., MOSKOWITZ R. A., FINK S. & SVEC K. H. (1972) Comprehensive care and psycho-social factors in rehabilitation in chronic rheumatoid arthritis: a controlled study. *Journal of Chronic Diseases,* **25,** 457–467.
[4] KATZ S., VIGNOS P. J. JR., MOSKOWITZ R. W., THOMPSON H. M. & SVEC K. H. (1968) Comprehensive outpatient care in rheumatoid arthritis. A controlled study. *Journal of the American Medical Association,* **206,** 1249.
[5] WRIGHT V. & OWEN S. (1976) The effect of rheumatoid arthritis on the social situation of housewives. *Rheumatology and Rehabilitation,* **15,** 156–160.
[6] MATTINGLY S. (1977) *Rehabilitation Today.* Update Publications, London.

Appendix A

COMMON LABORATORY TESTS USED IN THE RHEUMATOLOGICAL DISORDERS

Erythrocyte sedimentation rate (ESR)

A value above 20 mm/hour is regarded as abnormal.

It is an index of inflammation and tissue destruction.

The ESR is elevated in rheumatoid arthritis, systemic lupus erythematosus and polyarteritis nodosa.

When serial measurements of ESR are made it provides a useful guide to disease activity but when corticosteroids are used the test is of no significance because these drugs reduce the ESR. C-reactive protein is then a more valuable guide.

C-reactive protein

This is an abnormal serum globulin found in the presence of active inflammation and tissue damage.

Haemoglobin

The haemoglobin concentration is also related to disease activity. In rheumatoid arthritis anaemia is often present.

The sensitised sheep cell (SCAT) and latex fixation tests

Rheumatoid factor (RF) is an immunoglobulin M found in the serum of approximately 80% of patients with rheumatoid arthritis. Waaler discovered that the immunoglobulin reacted with the denatured gamma globulin of sheep red blood cells.

Latex fixation tests (LFT) are more sensitive but less specific than SCAT; the suspension of latex particles coated with denatured human gamma globulin aggregate in the presence of RF in the patient's serum.

These tests are used as diagnostic aids.

Positive IgM RF is found in 80% of patients with rheumatoid arthritis, 40% of those with systemic lupus erythematosus. It is negative in ankylosing spondylitis, Reiter's syndrome and osteoarthrosis.

LE cell test

This is a specific test for systemic lupus erythematosus, although occasionally a positive test may be found in rheumatoid arthritis and other connective tissue disorders. The test is performed *in vitro* and is positive when a specific globulin in the patient's serum reacts with the nuclei of cells. The polymorphs phagocytose the altered nuclear material and this can be identified in the polymorphonuclear leucocytes.

Antinuclear factor tests (ANF)

In patients with systemic lupus erythematosus the serum contains high titres of antibodies which react *in vitro* with cell nuclei. The antinuclear antibodies are detected by immunofluorescent techniques.

Urine analysis

PROTEINURIA

In rheumatoid arthritis may indicate amyloid disease, gold nephropathy or analgesic nephropathy. In collagen disorders presence of renal involvement.

URINE CHEMISTRY

Low urinary creatine is under 1000 mg per 24 hours in muscle diseases.

Muscle serum enzymes

CREATINE PHOSPHOKINASE (CPK)

This enzyme acts as a catalyst in the release of phsophate from creatine phosphate during muscle contraction. The enzyme occurs mainly in muscle. In diseases where muscle fibre degenerates the enzyme is found in the patient's serum.

Appendix B

DRUG THERAPY

Analgesics – Salicylates

Properties

Analgesic, antipyretic and mildly anti-inflammatory

Side effects

    Dyspepsia
    Gastroduodenal haemorrhage
    Tinnitus
    Disturbed acid-base balance
    Analgesic neuropathy

Anti-inflammatory

RAPIDLY ACTING

    Phenylbutazone + strong analgesic effect
    Indomethacin + analgesic effect
    Fenamates − mildly analgesic

Side effects

    Headache and vertigo

Dyspepsia
Peptic ulceration
Blood dyscrasias

SLOWLY ACTING

1. Gold injections – no analgesic effect

Side effects

Skin rashes
Mucosal ulceration
Diarrhoea
Albuminuria
*Gold is a sensitiser for ultraviolet light.

2. Anti-malarial drugs

Side effects

Irreversible retinitis

3. *Immuno-suppressive*
Azathioprine
D-penicillamine

Side effects

Leucopenia
Nausea, vomiting

Quickly acting, very powerful and strong analgesic effect

Systemic corticosteroids – prednisone

Side effects

Obesity
Moon face
Osteoporosis

Fluid retention
Muscle weakness
Ecchymoses
Masking effect on infection

Implications for physiotherapy

1. Over-stressing joints by excessive exercise – normally protected by pain-induced spasm.

2. Care in handling because of osteoporosis, e.g. in treating chest infection – ribs and thoracic vertebrae particularly vulnerable.

3. Attention for first signs of steroid-induced myopathy.

Index